Truth in
Nursing
Inquiry

To Marilynn J. Wood

Truth in Nursing Inquiry

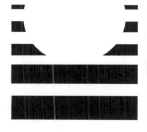

June F. Kikuchi
Helen Simmons
Donna Romyn
editors

SAGE Publications
International Educational and Professional Publisher
Thousand Oaks London New Delhi

For information address:

SAGE Publications, Inc.
2455 Teller Road
Thousand Oaks, California 91320
E-mail: order@sagepub.com

SAGE Publications Ltd.
6 Bonhill Street
London EC2A 4PU
United Kingdom

SAGE Publications India Pvt. Ltd.
M-32 Market
Greater Kailash I
New Delhi 110 048 India

Printed in the United States of America

Library of Congress Cataloging-in-Publication Data

Main entry under title:

Truth in nursing inquiry/editors, June F. Kikuchi, Helen Simmons,
    Donna Romyn.
        p. cm.
    Includes bibliographical references (p.) and index.
    ISBN 0-7619-0098-5 (cloth, alk. paper).—ISBN 0-7619-0099-3 (pbk.,
alk. paper).
    II. Simmons, Helen, 1927-   . III. Romyn, Donna.
    RT81.5.T785   1996   95-41742
    610.73'01—dc20

This book is printed on acid-free paper

96 97 98 99 00 10 9 8 7 6 5 4 3 2 1

Sage Production Editor: Diane S. Foster

Contents

Acknowledgments

We would like to thank and express our appreciation to all those who, in one form or another, helped make this volume possible. Particularly, we wish to thank the contributing authors for allowing us to include their papers in this volume and for working cooperatively with us as we proceeded through the editing process. We wish to renew our expression of gratitude to Dr. Marilynn Wood, Dean of the Faculty of Nursing at the University of Alberta, as well as to our faculty for their ongoing support of the Institute for Philosophical Nursing Research, under the auspices of which this book is being published.

We are indebted to Lucy Steen and Lynn Szoo for their expert secretarial assistance in the preparation of the book manuscript. Finally, our special thanks are extended to Christine Smedley, Assistant Editor at Sage Publications. Her support, cooperative spirit, and expert editorial advice made all the difference in bringing this volume to fruition.

Prologue:
Speaking of the Truth

The sole philosophy open to those who doubt the possibility of truth is absolute silence. (Maritain, 1962, p. 128)

Throughout the history of Western philosophy, the notion of truth has generated much discussion. Philosophers have argued, and continue to argue, about such issues as whether the kinds, measures, and sources of truth and the ways of attaining and expressing truth are one or many. Of course, one position on these issues has been that of the skeptic, denying the possibility of attaining truth at all. It is of concern that disciplined discussion of such issues, as they relate to nursing knowledge development, is rarely to be found in the nursing literature or at nursing research or theory conferences. By *disciplined discussion,* we mean discussion in which (a) the same interpretation of the question and subject matter at issue is held by all parties to the issue—that is, that they have come to terms; and (b) all answers are examined, in a reasonable manner, by all parties, with the aim of resolving the issue by working out apparent disagreements (Adler, 1958).

What could account for the lack of disciplined discussion of the matter of truth in nursing inquiry, and what would it take for such discussion to occur? It is not the purpose of this prologue to answer these questions but rather to invite those in nursing who are responsible for nursing knowledge development to take up disciplined discussion of them. To begin, let us consider what most, if not all, of us have witnessed at one time or another when the notion of pursuing truth in nursing is mentioned.

When the topic of pursuing truth in nursing is broached, most groups of nurses quickly divide into those who do and those who do not support that pursuit. Those who do not are usually quick to query, in a skeptical manner, "What is truth? How do we ascertain what is true or, for that matter, what truth is?" In the discussion that then ensues (without the parties having come to terms), typically more heat than light is generated. No notion, except perhaps for that of death or abortion, seems to generate such an emotional response as does that of truth. The discussion is almost always shut down by the declaration of skeptics who adamantly deny the possibility of knowing anything to be true because, in their view, there is no adequate criterion for determining the correctness of any judgment.

Unfortunately, the usual result of such discussions is that parties to the issue go away with their particular conceptions of truth and truth in nursing inquiry intact. They have not identified what is adequate or inadequate about their conceptions—in what respects these are true, erroneous, or false and in what respects they are or are not comprehensive. Over time, fruitless discussions of this sort take their toll. There comes a reluctance, on the part of many, to enter into any more discussions on the topic of truth. Of late, various related developments taking place both inside and outside the nursing discipline appear to be lending support to this reluctance.

The developments to which we are referring include the growing tendency (a) to adopt the notion that reality conforms to the mind; (b) to accept the idea that what is true, including conceptions of truth, is in the mind's eye of the beholder; and (c) to reject logical positivism because of its "failure" to allow us to come to know, and express what we know, about the lived experiences of events that humans encounter and the meanings they place on them. A full consideration of the factors leading up to each of these developments may help us understand better why we have moved away from discussions about truth, and the pursuit of truth itself, in nursing and what would be required of us to change this state of affairs. This is a task we leave our readers to undertake. However, so that this undertaking may start on common footing in the form of a common understanding of each development, a brief description of each development follows, beginning with that of conceiving of reality as conforming to the mind.

Whether reality conforms to the mind or the mind to reality is a perennial question that continues to challenge philosophers. How one answers it depends on how one orders the existence of reality and mind. If reality is assigned primacy and presumed to have existence before mind, then reality is taken to exist independent of the mind. The mind is said to seek factual knowledge about reality and to have attained it once its judgment is in conformity with reality and is coherent with other judgments held to be true. On the other hand, if the mind is assigned primacy and presumed to have existence before reality, then what is in the mind is imposed on reality, and reality is taken to be a reflection of what is in the mind. In this case, correspondence of the mind with reality is inappropriate as a measure of truth because reality does not exist independent of the mind. The mind then validates its ideas by using coherence or utility as a measure of truth (Adler, 1990; Bittle, 1936; Wallace, 1977).

Lately, in keeping with the thinking of such social scientists and/or philosophers as Gadamer, Guba, Lincoln, Heidegger, and Rorty, to name but a few, nurses in increasing numbers are no longer holding the position that the mind conforms to reality but rather are embracing the position that reality conforms to the mind. From this development has come the second position—a ready acceptance of the idea that what is true (including which conceptions of truth are true) is in the mind's eye of the beholder. In other words, truth is taken to be a matter of how we see things (or, in some cases, of how we prefer to see things) rather than of how things are, regardless of how we see them or would like them to be. Mitchell (1994) eloquently described this stance, vis-à-vis nursing science, basing her thinking in that of "Gadamerian hermeneutics" (p. 226).

In contemporary nursing, the adoption of the notion of worldviews is but one manifestation of the position that reality conforms to the mind and that truth is relative to persons. Nurses who have adopted the notion of worldviews can be heard to say that reality changes when one "puts on a different set of lenses." The upshot is that what is considered true according to one worldview may, at the same time, quite acceptably be considered false according to another because of the subjective way in which the world is viewed. Under these conditions, argumentation about what is true makes no sense whatsoever.

Finally, under the influence of the idea that reality conforms to the mind and truth is relative to persons, and of other similar ideas basic to the philosophies of phenomenology and existentialism, many have found logical positivism wanting. Logical positivism, with its perceived focus on the material, the objective, and that which is external to the self and also with its reliance on quantitative methods, is thought by a growing number of nurses to be inadequate and limiting. Many nurses believe that it does not allow for attaining and expressing what nurses need to know to practice humanely—that is, knowledge of patients/clients as autonomous beings, with their own developing perspectives and values that are true for them and therefore ought to be respected (Benner, 1994). To nurse in a humanistic manner, nurses have begun to seek new ways to attain and express patients/clients' perspectives of encountered health events and the meanings that these events have for them.

In many of the essays in this volume, the foregoing developments are evident; in the others, thinking quite contrary to these developments is apparent. Together, they are representative of the diversity of views about particular aspects of truth in nursing inquiry today. It is our hope that these essays will be helpful to readers as they consider the matter of truth in nursing inquiry and the lack of disciplined discussion of the same.

The essays themselves were invited by the Institute for Philosophical Nursing Research for its third biennial invitational conference on "Conceptions of Truth in Nursing Inquiry." This conference theme was selected because at the preceding second conference that was designed to uncover, through philosophical discussion, the sources of our opposing viewpoints on matters integral to developing a sound philosophy of nursing, a sustained reluctance to deal with the subject of truth per se was apparent.

The aim in bringing this collection of essays to publication is twofold: (a) to bring into the open, for discussion, the prevailing conceptions of truth in nursing inquiry—the diversity of conceptions related to the kinds, measures, and expressions of truth in nursing inquiry; and (b) to stimulate disciplined discussion of the significance of the pursuit of truth for nursing knowledge development and the consequences of continuing to avoid speaking of truth, in all its dimensions.

The book is divided into three parts. Part I is devoted to the topic of kinds of truth in nursing inquiry, Part II to measures of truth in nursing inquiry, and Part III to expressions of truth in nursing inquiry. As readers will soon discover, this division is rather arbitrary. The topics are related; consequently various aspects of them appear, in one form or another, in many of the essays. The primary emphasis of each essay determined its placement in a particular part of the book.

Introductions to each part of the book are followed by guiding questions that are in no way meant as a test of knowledge. They are designed to lay bare some of the questions behind the essays and to help readers get the most out of each author's philosophical perspective on a topic intimately related to truth in nursing inquiry. In the last analysis, they are designed to assist readers in making up their own minds on the topic at hand.

If students and seasoned scholars feel at all called upon to philosophize about truth in nursing inquiry because of the essays presented here, we as editors will regard the publication as a work worth having done.

References

Adler, M. J. (1958). *The idea of freedom: Vol. 1. A dialectical examination of the conception of freedom*. Garden City, NY: Doubleday.

Adler, M. J. (1990). *Intellect: Mind over matter*. New York: Macmillan.

Benner, P. (Ed.). (1994). *Interpretive phenomenology*. Newbury Park, CA: Sage.

Bittle, C. (1936). *Reality and the mind*. New York: Bruce.

Maritain, J. (1962). *An introduction to philosophy* (E. I. Watkin, Trans.). New York: Sheed & Ward.

Mitchell, G. J. (1994). Discipline-specific inquiry: The hermeneutics of theory-guided nursing research. *Nursing Outlook, 42*, 224-228.

Wallace, W. A. (1977). *The elements of philosophy*. New York: Alba House.

PART I

Kinds of Truth
in Nursing Inquiry

When nurses engage in nursing research, it is clear that they are seeking knowledge. In speaking of the aim of their endeavors, they inevitably refer to the development of nursing's body of knowledge. Also, many declare, following the thinking of Carper (1978), that utilization of multiple ways of knowing is necessary to develop nursing knowledge. But amidst all this talk about nursing knowledge and ways of knowing in nursing, mention of the word *truth* is conspicuously absent.

Whether truth is being sought, and if so what *kind,* is most often left unstated by nurse researchers. Why? Is it because truth is regarded as truth and that is all there is to it? Is it because knowledge is thought to have nothing to do with truth and falsity? Is it that truth, not to mention different kinds of truth, is thought to be unattainable? Or is it that different degrees of truth are thought to exist but not different kinds?

Possible explanations for the apparent neglect of truth by nurse researchers are all but limitless. Nonetheless, to say that truth is (or is not) attainable, that knowledge has something (or nothing) to do with truth and falsity, or that there is (or is not) more than one kind of truth has ramifications for any effort at developing nursing's body of knowledge. For example, if we say that truth is unattainable and that knowledge has nothing to do with truth and falsity, we are faced with the question "What, then, constitutes the body of nursing knowledge that we are purporting to develop?" Is not the only possible answer to this question "mere opinion"? And to say that there is only one kind of truth (e.g., the scientific) leaves nurses knowing their world from only that one perspective and not seeking truths of any other kind, such as philosophical or historical truths, in relation to the nurse's world.

Because of the need to confront the problem of whether truth is attainable at all in nursing inquiry and, if so, whether different kinds of truth exist, Part I of this volume is devoted to the topic of kinds of truth in nursing inquiry. In Chapter 1, Kikuchi and Simmons examine the notion of "the whole truth" and the role of the logic of truth and of truth-relevant distinctions in the development of nursing's body of knowledge. In Chapter 2, Holden identifies a set of criteria, in the form of nursing competencies, for identifying the possession (existence) of four levels (or kinds) of nursing knowledge that, resulting from rational and empirical thought, fall into the realm of truth as opposed to that of opinion. In Chapter 3, Johnson, focusing more specifically on practical nursing knowledge, draws a definite distinction between speculative and prescriptive truth in discussing the place of prescriptive truths in nursing art.

Reference

Carper, B. (1978). Fundamental patterns of knowing in nursing. *Advances in Nursing Science, 1*(1), 13-23.

Guiding Questions:
Making up Your Own Mind

What criterion (or criteria) ought to be used in nursing inquiry to determine whether a nursing proposition is true or false?

If one espouses an idealist nursing philosophy (i.e., holds that the most important element in the nature of reality is the mind), why is it necessary to merge the questions (a) What is truth? and (b) By what means can we determine if this or that proposition is true?

Can nursing escape making exclusionary claims in the course of developing its body of knowledge?

Are the different truths sought in nursing inquiry different in degree or different in kind?

Under the philosophy that nothing is static and discontinuous in nature but rather that all is dynamic and continuous, is it logically congruent to speak of different kinds of truth?

Are the different kinds of truth in nursing inquiry related to each other?

Are there only speculative nursing truths, only practical nursing truths, or both? If both, how are speculative nursing truths related to practical nursing truths? How are speculative nursing truths related to the speculative truths of other disciplines?

Are the rules of nursing art one kind of nursing truth? If so, are they to be found in the body of nursing knowledge?

Is it appropriate to use the word *truth* in relation to nursing competencies? Does "know-how" fall into the realm of truth?

What kind of truth is attainable in the particular case?

CHAPTER 1

The Whole Truth and Progress in Nursing Knowledge Development

JUNE F. KIKUCHI
HELEN SIMMONS

In contemporary philosophical nursing discourse, relatively little time and energy have been devoted to the topic of truth per se. It is a foregone conclusion, however, that nurses, in their undertakings as inquirers, are invested not in pursuing falsity but rather in pursuing its opposite, truth. In addition, they do claim *cognitive status* for their theories—that is, they aspire to be developing nursing knowledge and so, knowingly or not, subject their products to the criteria of truth and falsity. In so doing, they are bound by the logic of truth, in which the irrefragable unity of truth or the whole truth is presupposed.

The title of this chapter is meant to imply that the relationship between the whole truth and the possibility of making progress in nursing knowledge development is an intimate one. The motive force behind the chapter is the apprehension that if in our efforts to develop nursing knowledge we ignore the whole truth and thereby the logical considerations that underlie engagement in the pursuit of truth, we do so at nursing's peril. Under such conditions, the body of nursing knowledge required to guide nursing practice will, in effect, be stillborn. Our purpose in writing this chapter is to draw attention to that fact. The chapter begins with a brief description of the problem, proceeds through a descriptive definition of *the whole truth* to the conditions under which progress toward the whole truth within (and outside) the nursing discipline may be made, and concludes with the consequences for progress in nursing knowledge development of not making or maintaining certain truth-relevant distinctions.

The Problem

The problem, as we see it, regarding the whole truth and nursing knowledge development is that nurse scholars, while aspiring to develop nursing knowledge or simply to make cognitive claims for their beliefs and theories, are increasingly (wittingly or not) ignoring the whole truth and, related to it, certain truth-relevant distinctions. In doing so, they are violating the *logic of truth:* the laws, principles, and rules of logic that one must follow in the pursuit of truth. In violating these elements, particularly the principle of noncontradiction, they embrace and invite undisputed contrary/contradictory propositions into the body of nursing knowledge. Progress in nursing knowledge development is thereby rendered a logical impossibility because epistemological progress presupposes the principle of noncontradiction. This principle, in its ontological form, states that a thing cannot both be and not be at the same time. As a logical principle, it states that the truth of the same proposition cannot, at the same time, be both affirmed and denied (Brubacher, 1957; Wallace, 1977).

The Whole Truth

The whole truth (and nothing but) is the ideal goal of the pursuit of truth—that is, the commitment to a never-ending endeavor of getting to *know* all that is *knowable* In other words, the pursuit of truth (of which the whole truth is the goal) is really the pursuit of knowledge. When we say we "know" something, we mean we have grasped the truth about it. To speak of "true knowledge" is to be redundant; to speak of "false knowledge" is to be contradictory (Adler, 1981, p. 49). The pursuit of truth goes on only in the realm of doubt, where truth is mingled with error.[1]

There are two senses of *whole* (in "the whole truth") that must be accommodated if we are to retain any hope of developing a body of nursing knowledge adequate to guide nursing practice: (a) the sense in which *whole* means all—all the different kinds of truth that exist— and (b) the sense in which *whole* refers to the quality of "unity" or "oneness" of truth.

In the first sense of *whole*, one thinks of all the qualifying adjectives or predicates applied to the subject of truth: for example, natural and supernatural, objective and subjective, logical or factual and poetical,[2] absolute and probable, formal and informal. Failing to make or maintain such distinctions and to acknowledge the existence of all the different kinds of truth leads to all sorts of folly in our attempts to develop nursing knowledge—a point to be elaborated upon later in this chapter.

In the second sense of *whole*, we think of Aquinas's (1952) and, more latterly, of Newman's (1852/1915) conception of truth as one comprehensive, all-embracing *unity* with *diverse* parts—a unity in the sense that all parts making up the whole, no matter how diverse, are coherent and compatible. They are coherent in that they are parts in one and the same whole of the mind's realm of thought, and they are compatible in that one part does not conflict with any of the other parts of the whole. The *unity* of truth is due to the logic of truth, which is the same across formal branches of knowledge and applies to all propositions that are subject to contradiction. The *diversity* of the parts is due to the different objects focused on, the different methods of discovery, and the different sources in experience that ground the different formal branches of knowledge (Adler, 1990b, pp. 17, 22-27, 142).

NURSING AND
THE WHOLE OF TRUTH

All the formal disciplines or branches of knowledge (the empirical sciences, philosophy, history, and mathematics) claim logical or factual truth for their propositions, whether descriptive or prescriptive. Nursing as a discipline (as one of the sciences) is simply one component in the whole of truth, and it, like every other part, is bound by the logic of truth and "must have coherence and be compatible with all the other parts of the whole. . . . *[That much] is what is required by the logic of truth in terms of the unity of truth* [italics added]" (Adler, 1990b, p. 27). Bound by the logic of truth, nursing as a discipline is obligated to monitor whether its propositions cohere and are compatible with propositions known to be true inside and outside the discipline. When its propositions conflict with what is known to be true, they cannot simply be left undisputed.

All the formal disciplines claiming logical truth hold, as *universally* applicable, the notion that (following sufficient investigation and weighing of the evidence and/or reasons) whatever is inconsistent or incompatible with agreed-upon truths at a given time must be regarded as false. This consequence is a significant extension of the principle of noncontradiction. The disproof of either a descriptive or a prescriptive proposition can be accomplished by the proof of its contrary or of its contradictory.[3] According to the logic of truth, two contradictory propositions cannot both be true—one must be true, the other false. And of two contrary propositions, both cannot be true, but both may be false (Brubacher, 1957). With every nursing proposition we put forward, we must first decide whether we are making a cognitive claim and, if so, whether, as far as we know, it is coherent and compatible with the rest of the whole of truth. If we do less, we fail to meet our moral obligation to our own and other disciplines in the pursuit of truth.

Making Progress in
the Pursuit of Truth

When we speak of making progress in the pursuit of truth within a discipline such as nursing, we really are committing ourselves to resolving our differences of opinion about which of our judgments are true and to what degree. A reasonable commitment is to seek and attain enough agreement or unity on the truth of this or that matter to allow us to move on to other unresolved differences. Unity to this extent is required to attain the object of nursing's inquiry (nursing truths) and, in turn, the end goal of nursing practice.

Being bound by the logic of truth, we are not allowed the luxury (some would say "the inaneness") of agreeing to disagree. Progress in any discipline depends on the working out of disagreements: testing and weighing the evidence and/or reasons for and against various propositions. Out of our controversies and disagreements come the research studies, investigations, and arguments by which disputes at the expanding edge of the whole truth can be resolved and temporarily agreed-upon truths come by. Agreed-upon truths are those in the realm of doubt where our judgments lack certitude but are temporarily undisputed by experts competent to judge—scientists, philosophers, mathematicians, and historians in their own fields of inquiry (Adler, 1981, p. 57).

In the realm of doubt, the means by which we come closer to the whole truth, and nothing but, include the addition of newly discovered truths; the replacement of less comprehensive formulations with more comprehensive ones; the discovery and rectification of errors; and the discarding of hypotheses, generalizations, and theories that have been shown to be false by the discovery of contrary instances (Adler, 1981, pp. 49-50, 56-57; Schlotfeldt, 1988). It is important to note that if we admit that we can carry out any one of these activities, we admit the possibility of making *progress* in our grasp of the truth; and, if we admit such a possibility in the various disciplines, we admit the unity of truth.

To recapitulate, making progress in nursing knowledge development plainly and simply depends upon nurse inquirers' acknowledging that truth is all of a piece—one indisputable whole that does not admit of contraries or contradictions—and that as long as we claim cognitive status for our propositions, we cannot escape the logic of truth and its consequences. We cannot make progress toward the whole truth within the nursing discipline or beyond it if we embrace and invite contrary/contradictory propositions, undisputed, into the body of nursing knowledge. For example, propositions such as "the end goal of nursing is adaptation" and "the end goal of nursing is consciousness raising" cannot be left undisputed if we claim to be developing knowledge. Using appropriate means, we must determine which of such putative truths, if any, are true to a defensible degree and similarly which, if any, are false.

If we keep in mind these notions related to the whole truth or unity of truth, it will be easier to understand how people might unwittingly or even defiantly introduce undisputed, logically incompatible propositions—contrary/contradictory propositions—into the body of nursing knowledge. Those who do so defiantly are most apt to be those who opine that there is no such thing as objective truth and that contradiction is therefore irrelevant. By so dismissing the principle of noncontradiction and with it the unity or wholeness of truth, they avoid the consequence of claiming logical truth for the nursing discipline—the obligation to regard as false whatever is inconsistent or incompatible with truths agreed upon at a given time. The only other means by which this obligation can be avoided is to regard the discipline as making no cognitive claims whatsoever but as being simply a matter of taste (Adler, 1990b). In either case, we abort the possibility of one proposition challenging another (inside the whole of nursing truth or between it and the rest of the whole of truth)—that is, the possibility of the genuine disagreement (and the subsequent agreement) required for progress in nursing knowledge development.

One glaring piece of evidence that these means of avoidance are presently operative in nursing inquiry is the adoption by many nurses of the notion of worldviews (e.g., see Fawcett, 1993). Worldviews make absolutely no claim of being true and so avoid the logic of truth with regard to exclusionary claims.[4] Similarly, the contemporaneously popular practice among nurse scholars (e.g., Newman, 1990; Stevens Barnum, 1994) of rejecting disjunctions (dichotomies) and declaring that certain frameworks are so distinctive that their products cannot be challenged from outside their particular framework (e.g., Fawcett,

1995) seems to us to be averroistic thinking (i.e., intellectual compart-mentalizing) of the most divisive sort. The implicit (and illicit) assump-tion, apparently, is that truth is not all of a piece and that the logic of truth does not apply (where, in fact, it does). The negative conse-quences for the pursuit of the whole of truth and for nursing knowl-edge development seem clear.

Because the logic of truth, in terms of the irrefragable unity of truth, will not admit of contrary/contradictory propositions existing side by side, logically incompatible nursing propositions introduced into the body of nursing knowledge call for resolution or expulsion. The alternative is to abandon the pursuit of truth and the possibility of attaining a body of nursing knowledge consisting of a coherent and compatible set of propositions in favor of compiling an endless collection of nonexclusionary propositions—propositions reflective of temperamental and emotional predilections, prejudices, and pref-erences. Needless to say, the latter are unarguable matters of taste. In the realm of taste, where the logic of truth does not apply, diversity, not unity, is the acceptable and desirable state of affairs. There, any attempt at progress in terms of coherence or compatibility is an irrelevant, if not a ridiculous, aspiration.

The undisputed introduction of logically incompatible propositions into the body of nursing knowledge is most often due to a failure to make or maintain one or another very important truth-relevant dis-tinction. The distinctions of consequence are those (a) among all the diverse parts in the whole of the truth we can come to know or (b) among the various aspects of reality the truth of which is being pursued. If a significant number of nurse scholars were to ignore these distinctions *on a sustained basis,* any attempt at progress in nursing knowledge develop-ment would be rendered a logical impossibility. We contend that various philosophical notions being adopted in nursing harbor that likelihood.

Some Truth-Relevant Distinctions

With the adoption in nursing of notions of dynamism, holism, and continuity has come rejection of the practice of distinguishing between entities (i.e., noting essential differences between them) and treating them as separate entities in their own right. This rejection is evident in the growing tendency, among nurse scholars, neither to make nor to maintain, or to blur, certain truth-relevant distinctions, such as those between subjective and objective truth, probable and absolute truth, logical or factual and poetical truth, descriptive and prescriptive truth, and truth and taste. Let us examine each of these distinctions in turn, beginning with the one between subjective and objective truth.

SUBJECTIVE AND OBJECTIVE TRUTH

According to Adler (1981), the subjective aspect of truth can be distinguished from the objective in that the subjective aspect "lies in the claim that the individual makes for the veracity of his judgement [whereas] the objective aspect lies in the agreement or correspondence between what an individual believes or opines and the reality about which he is making a judgement when he holds a certain belief or opinion" (p. 42). The objective and subjective aspects of truth actually supplement each other (Adler, 1990b, pp. 25, 127).

In the works of nurse phenomenologists/existentialists (e.g., see Cody, 1993, 1994; Smith, 1991), there appears to be a reluctance to admit the objective aspect of truth and a tendency to focus solely on the subjective aspect. Every individual's opinion is then considered to be "true." Presumably, the belief that the nature of reality is not independent of the human mind lies behind this stance. The upshot, for our discipline, of not maintaining a distinction between the subjective and objective aspects of truth and of focusing only on the subjective aspect is significant. We are left with no legitimate basis for resolving differences of opinion and with no means by which to replace errors and falsities with truths. Nursing's body of knowledge can thus expand to infinity with ever-changing nonexclusionary propositions, some (or all) of which may be contrary to each other or to what has been established as true in other parts of the whole of truth. Can the discipline of nursing survive such uncorrected and unrestrained subjectivism? What measure could we possibly call upon to assess whether the discipline is making progress?

PROBABLE AND ABSOLUTE TRUTH

A second distinction that tends to be blurred is that between probable and absolute truth. Most of our judgments fall within the shadow of doubt (the realm of doubt or of the probable rather than the realm of certitude) and are therefore subject to change and correction.[5] This becomes apparent only when the distinction between probable and absolute truth is acknowledged.

When nurse inquirers fail to distinguish between probable truth and absolute truth, their common sense balks at the notion of pursuing truth. The claim of those who do distinguish between probable and absolute truth—that some propositions are true beyond a shadow of a doubt (absolute truth), some are true beyond a reasonable doubt or supported by a preponderance of evidence and reason (probable truth), and some make no claim on truth whatsoever—becomes replaced, in the minds of those who do not make this distinction, with the repugnant claim that all truth is absolute. Consequently the pursuit of truth is interpreted by the latter as a wild-goose chase for one certain truth—*the* Truth. Hence such inquirers fall into absolute skepticism and give up altogether on the notion that truth is attainable. It is no wonder that they find, in this confusion, a clear invitation to substitute the pursuit of personal predilections, preferences, and unsupported prejudices (with all their inherent diversity) for what they regard as the hopeless pursuit of "one absolute truth."

LOGICAL AND POETICAL TRUTH

Another distinction that a number of nurse theorists tend not to make or maintain, of late, is that between logical and poetical truth. The line that divides the actual from the possible also divides logical truth from poetical truth. Logical truth is attributable to propositions that are about the actual and are therefore subject to contradiction. The products to which poetical truth applies are about the possible and are therefore *not* subject to contradiction—they are in no way incompatible with each other and are not subject to the logic of truth (Adler, 1990b, pp. 10-11).

The personal stories or narratives of patients/clients, recently being appealed to by nurse scholars such as Gadow (1990) and Sandelowski (1991) as a source of nursing truths, would appear to fall into the realm of poetical truth in that all the stories are apparently viewed as possible and true. For example, two "opposite" renditions of what it means to have a heart attack are not seen as incompatible and requiring resolution—both are accepted as true. Yet only the most popular rendition (the one told by most of the storytellers) seems to be manifest in the themes (categories) and theory that are eventually developed (e.g., see Diekelmann, 1993; Meleis, Arruda, Lane, & Bernal, 1994). Elimination of the "unpopular" renditions would seem to signify that the stories are viewed as belonging to the logical, rather than the poetical, realm. We contend that the apparent slippage in thought here is a function of losing sight of the line that divides the actual from the possible, the logical from the poetical.

DESCRIPTIVE AND PRESCRIPTIVE TRUTH

A further important distinction that nurses in increasing numbers are failing to make—one leading to additional confusion and the ready introduction of logically incompatible propositions into the body of nursing knowledge—is that between descriptive and prescriptive truth. The significance of making this distinction is doubly important because not making it transports nursing practice, as concerned with the common good and justice, out of the realm of truth into the realm of taste—a further distinction to which we will return in a moment.

If the distinction is not drawn between descriptive truth (truth about "what is") and prescriptive truth (truth about "what ought to be done"), it becomes very easy to treat values or ethics—our conceptualizations of "the good"—as if they were noncognitive matters, matters of taste or preference (e.g., see Cody, 1993). Making this distinction requires that we solve the problem raised by Hume in the 18th century.

Hume made the point that from factual knowledge of what is, we cannot infer a single true proposition about what ought to be done. Humean skepticism (that there is no criterion for the establishment of the truth of "oughts") is apparent today in the form of noncognitive or emotive ethics in which "oughts" are thought to be neither true nor false. Hume, like many modern and contemporary philosophers, failed to see that Aristotle had provided a solution to the problem of the criterion for practical truth, namely, right desire.[6] Aristotle demonstrated that an inference about "oughts" could be drawn from an argument containing (a) the self-evidently true prescriptive premise— the first principle of moral philosophy, namely, that we ought to desire what is really good for us and only that (i.e., right desire)—or a prescriptive premise derived therefrom (as the major premise) and (b) a descriptive premise in the form of a factual truth about human nature (as the minor premise) that identifies what is really good for human beings in terms of inherent human desires or natural needs (Adler, 1981, 1990b).

Because an adequate solution to the problem raised by Hume has been available to us since antiquity, it behooves us to get on with recognizing that prescriptions do possess truth but not in the same way that descriptive propositions do: That is, they possess truth through conformity with right desire rather than with "what is." With this recognition, "oughts" are seen for what they are—cognitive matters, arguable and applicable to all by way of universal standards of moral behavior. The availability of such standards, it should be remarked, makes possible the cooperative pursuit of justice and the common good by everyone.

TRUTH AND TASTE

A final distinction that tends to be ignored (particularly by those educated in the idealist philosophy)[7] has been referred to, in passing, earlier in this chapter. It is that between truth and taste. Recall that the logic of truth does not apply to matters of taste but does apply to matters of truth; tastes or preferences are nonexclusionary and unarguable, and diversity is the acceptable and desirable state of affairs in the realm of taste.

By idealists, matters of truth are often treated as matters of taste or preference. Consequently, of matters of truth, they say, for example, "That may be true for you, but it's not for me." Consistent with their failure to make or maintain the distinction between truth and taste and with their presupposition that there is no reality independent of the human mind, they set diversity of thought as the *preferred* end goal or object of nursing inquiry (e.g., Barrett, 1992; Stevens Barnum, 1994). In doing so, they deny not only the wholeness or unity of nursing truth as constituting one part in the whole of truth proper but also, perhaps without realizing it, the need for an organized body (unity) of nursing knowledge. These denials entail relinquishing the notion of nursing as a discipline and the possibility of nurses meeting their moral obligation as scholars to develop knowledge that is coherent and compatible with the whole of human knowledge. These are serious consequences.

Conclusion

If nurse scholars aspire to develop an organized body of nursing knowledge, they cannot escape the logic of truth or the necessity of making certain truth-relevant distinctions. Should they attempt to escape, they must abandon any hope of progress being made in the nursing discipline. They must abandon the pursuit of truth (and with it the whole or unity of truth) and thereby plunge nursing inquiry into a welter of personal predilections, preferences, and prejudices. A grim trade-off indeed!

Notes

1. The pursuit of truth does not go on in the realm of certitude nor in the realm of taste, for in both of those realms error, as such, does not exist as an issue to be reckoned with.

2. By virtue of the fact that the principle of noncontradiction is an ontological principle as well as a logical principle, factual and logical truths coincide (Adler, 1990b). Poetical truths are subject not to the logic of truth but rather to the logic of preference (Adler, 1990b; VonWright, 1963). "The line that divides fact from fiction and fantasy, divides logical from poetical truth" (Adler, 1990b, p. 126).

3. In contemporary times, philosophers and others refer to contraries and contradictories as weak and strong disjunctions, respectively (Adler, 1990b).

4. An exclusionary claim is one that holds that if this particular proposition is correctly judged to be true, then *all* judgments to the contrary are false—no matter

whether the proposition is a mathematical theorem, a scientific generalization, a philosophical principle, or a religious article of faith (Adler, 1990b).

5. Conceptualizations of truth in their deceptive aspects should persuade us of the fallibility of the human mind and should restrain us from claiming certitude, finality, and incorrigibility for our judgments about what is true because they obviously are subject to doubt, change, and correction (Adler, 1981). The problem of the correctness of our judgments is the problem of the criterion (Chisholm, 1973).

6. In what follows, only right desire and practical thinking as they pertain to the sphere of doing (the moral and the political) are considered. In the sphere of making (the artistic), practical thinking would also entail drawing a prescriptive inference from a prescriptively true premise and a descriptively true premise (Adler, 1990a). However, in the sphere of making, right desire consists of desiring as one ought for the good of the work to be made as opposed to the good of human beings, as is the case in the sphere of doing (Maritain, 1970).

7. By the *idealist philosophy* is meant, here, the metaphysical theory that holds that the most important element in the nature of reality is the mind.

References

Adler, M. J. (1981). *Six great ideas*. New York: Macmillan.

Adler, M. J. (1990a). *Intellect: Mind over matter*. New York: Macmillan.

Adler, M. J. (1990b). *Truth in religion: The plurality of religions and the unity of truth*. New York: Macmillan.

Aquinas, T. (1952). *The summa theologica* (Fathers of the Dominican Province, Trans.). In R. M. Hutchins (Ed.), *Great books of the Western world* (Vol. 19, pp. 3-826). Chicago: Encyclopaedia Brittanica.

Barrett, E. A. (1992). Diversity reigns: Response to Northrup. *Nursing Science Quarterly, 5*(4), 155-157.

Brubacher, A. H. (1957). *Introduction to logic*. New York: Appleton-Century-Crofts.

Chisholm, R. M. (1973). *The problem of the criterion*. Milwaukee, WI: Marquette University Press.

Cody, W. K. (1993). Norms and nursing science: A question of values. *Nursing Science Quarterly, 6*(3), 110-112.

Cody, W. K. (1994). Nursing theory-guided practice: What it is and what it is not. *Nursing Science Quarterly, 7*(4), 144-145.

Diekelmann, N. L. (1993). Behavioral pedagogy: A Heideggerian hermeneutical analysis of the lived experiences of students and teachers in baccalaureate nursing education. *Journal of Nursing Education, 32*(6), 245-250.

Fawcett, J. (1993). From a plethora of paradigms to parsimony in worldviews. *Nursing Science Quarterly, 6*(2), 56-58.

Fawcett, J. (1995). *Analysis and evaluation of conceptual models of nursing* (3rd ed.). Philadelphia: F. A. Davis.

Gadow, S. (1990, October). *Beyond dualism: The dialectic of caring and knowing*. Paper presented at the conference, "The Care-Justice Puzzle: Education for Ethical Nursing Practice," Minneapolis.

Maritain, J. (1970). Art as a virtue of the practical intellect. In M. Weitz (Ed.), *Problems in aesthetics* (pp. 76-92). London: Macmillan.

Meleis, A. I., Arruda, E. N., Lane, S., & Bernal, P. (1994). Veiled, voluminous, and devalued: Narrative stories about low-income from Brazil, Egypt, and Columbia. *Advances in Nursing Science, 17*(2), 1-15.

Newman, J. H. (1915). *On the scope and nature of university education.* London: Dent & Son. (Original work published 1852)

Newman, M. A. (1990). Newman's theory of health as praxis. *Nursing Science Quarterly, 3*(1), 37-41.

Sandelowski, M. (1991). Telling stories: Narrative approaches in qualitative research. *Image, 23*(3), 161-166.

Schlotfeldt, R. (1988). Structuring nursing knowledge: A priority for creating nursing's future. *Nursing Science Quarterly, 1*(1), 35-38.

Smith, M. C. (1991). Existential-phenomenological foundations in nursing: A discussion of differences. *Nursing Science Quarterly, 4*(1), 5-6.

Stevens Barnum, B. J. (1994). *Nursing theory: Analysis, application, evaluation* (4th ed.). Philadelphia: J. B. Lippincott.

VonWright, G. H. (1963). *The logic of preference.* Edinburgh: Edinburgh University Press.

Wallace, W. A. (1977). *The elements of philosophy.* New York: Alba House.

CHAPTER 2

Nursing Knowledge: The Problem of the Criterion

ROBYN J. HOLDEN

Knowledge can be divided into two broad categories: practical and propositional. Practical knowledge is demonstrated in the mastery of psychomotor skills, whereas propositional knowledge is expressed in truth-functional sentences in which the proposition contained there can be demonstrated to be either true or false. Such propositions may convey either necessary truths or contingent truths. It is the elucidation of propositional knowledge that remains central to the philosophical debate in epistemology.

Essentially, the problem in epistemology is to answer two fundamental questions: "What counts as knowledge?" and "How does one know that what one knows is true?" In other words, how can one distinguish between knowledge and true opinion or belief? For example, I may strongly believe that God exists and even believe I have good independent grounds for believing that God exists, but such belief cannot count as knowledge because the truth of the belief cannot

19

be indisputably established in the same way that a mathematical or empirical truth can be indisputably established. Similarly, a man in the Middle Ages may have held fast to the controversial opinion that the earth was round. The man's opinion was in fact true, but unless he possessed the mathematical genius of Galileo, he would not have been able to demonstrate the truth of his belief. Therefore his true opinion would not count as genuine knowledge.

Rather than enter the philosophical debate with respect to identifying the hallmarks of a true, justified belief, about which philosophical volumes have been written, I shall instead turn my attention to the problem at hand: establishing the criteria for identifying nursing knowledge. In this chapter, I shall do so by first outlining the epistemological problem as initially addressed by Plato. I shall then draw a distinction between the rationalist position and the position later advanced by the empiricists. Although the intricacies of the philosophical debate between rationalism and empiricism will be circumvented, a new schema of various levels of knowledge will be presented and its relationship to nursing knowledge demonstrated. Finally, a set of criteria reflective of nursing knowledge will be presented, in the form of nursing competencies, and its merit deliberated. Let me begin by grounding the discussion in its historical context. To this end, I shall turn to Plato.

Epistemology:
The Historical Context

The problem of knowledge, along with the associated problem of certainty, is one that has plagued philosophy since the time of the early Greeks. Plato (1987) addressed this problem in *The Republic,* in which he articulated his theory of the Forms. In *The Republic,* he identified two levels of reality: that of essence and that of appearance. True knowledge, he claimed, can be attained only by fully comprehending the essence of a thing; knowledge derived from the realm of appearance has a secondary epistemological status. The realm of appearance is that level of reality apprehended by the senses through direct empirical experience. According to Plato, this level of reality—that is, the concrete, contingent world—is mistakenly identified as the real world. In contrast, the essence or the form of a thing is nonmaterial, lacks spatiotemporal location, and represents the ideal embodiment of all that exists in the world of appearance. Thus a form is an abstraction of a concrete particular and, as such, cannot be experienced through the senses but rather is experienced through the intellect alone. Plato was convinced, therefore, that forms are the only true reality from which all true knowledge is derived.[1]

To illustrate his position, Plato employed the analogy of the cave in Part 7, Book 7, of *The Republic*. He invited the reader to imagine people inhabiting a cave who had their backs always turned toward the sun so that only the shadows of the concrete world were visible on the far wall of the cave. Thus the passing shadows were mistaken by the people for the real world. Plato claimed that what is taken by us to be the real world—namely, concrete material reality—is equivalent to the passing shadows. However, he claimed that philosophers, with their superior intellect, are capable of seeing beyond the world of appearance. Through it, they gain entry into Plato's "ideal world" of nonthings, that is, the world of essence or forms.

Plato (1987) argued throughout *The Republic* that the realm of the nonmaterial or "ideal" is of higher ontological status than that of the material or the "real." The former is the object of true knowledge; the latter yields only mere opinion. Thus a philosopher must possess a passion for wisdom, the satisfaction of which depends on his capacity to draw distinctions between true knowledge (wisdom), mere opinion, and ignorance. Knowledge, according to Plato, "is related to what is, and ignorance necessarily to what is not" (477b). After some elaborate discussion, he concluded that opinion must mediate between knowledge and ignorance—between what is and what is not.

For Plato (1987), to be in possession of true knowledge is to see beauty-in-itself, goodness-in-itself, or justice-in-itself. He stated,

> Those then who have eyes for the multiplicity of beautiful things and just acts, and so on, but are unable, even with another to guide them, to see beauty itself, and justice itself, may be said in all cases to have opinion, but cannot be said to know any of the things they hold opinions about. (479e)

He then claimed that only "those who have eyes for the eternal, unchanging things" (479c) do possess true knowledge. Indeed, throughout Part 7 of *The Republic*, constant reference is made to this "eternal reality." For example, Plato stated that "one trait in the philosopher's character we can assume is his love for any branch of learning that reveals eternal reality, the realm unaffected by the vicissitudes of change and decay" (485b).

Plato (1987) offered two analogies to convey more clearly his conception of eternal reality. One, the "Sun Analogy" (Figure 2.1), draws a distinction between the "visible world" and the "intelligible world." In this analogy, the visible world is the world of appearance and the object of opinion; the intelligible world is the world of essence and the object of knowledge. "Particulars are the objects of sight but not intelligence, while forms are the objects of intelligence but not of sight" (507b). However, sight and seeing are existentially dependent on light, without which vision is impossible. Similarly, knowledge is existentially dependent on the accurate apprehension of truth and reality by the mind's eye—the intellect.

From the "Sun Analogy," Plato (1987) proceeded to another analogy, the "Divided-Line Analogy" (Figure 2.2). In this analogy, he began with the epistemological distinction between knowledge *(epistémé)* and opinion *(doxa)*. According to Plato, intelligence and mathematical reasoning are subclasses of knowledge, both of which permit apprehension of the forms that constitute the intelligible realm. On the other hand, opinion arises from belief and illusion, belief being associated with physical things and illusion with shadows and images. Both are of the visible (physical) realm.

From the above schema, it can be seen that the epistemological status of opinion is such that it relies on observation of the physical world for its formulations, whereas the epistemological status of knowledge is such that it relies, not on empirical observation, but on the intellect alone. In this account, forms embrace necessary truths, theorems, maxims, definitions, and universals, all of which are abstract entities apprehended solely by the intellect. The forms lack spatiotemporal location; they are nonmaterial, conceptual ideas, the comprehension of which is a precondition for becoming a philosopher. However, Plato was not suggesting that philosophers must be en-

Visible World	Intelligible World
The Sun	The Good
Source of growth and light, which gives visibility to objects of sense and the power of seeing to the eye	Source of reality and truth, which gives intelligibility to objects of thought and the power of knowing to the mind
The faculty of sight	The faculty of knowledge

Figure 2.1. Sun Analogy

SOURCE: Adapted with permission of Penguin Books Ltd. from *The Republic* by Plato, translated by Desmond Lee (Penguin Classics, 1935; second revised edition, 1987, p. 306). Copyright © H. D. P. Lee, 1953, 1974, 1987.

dowed with special, mystical, psychical powers capable of "seeing" what is hidden from lesser mortals. Rather, he emphasized repeatedly that philosophers must demonstrate a superior intellect, by which they

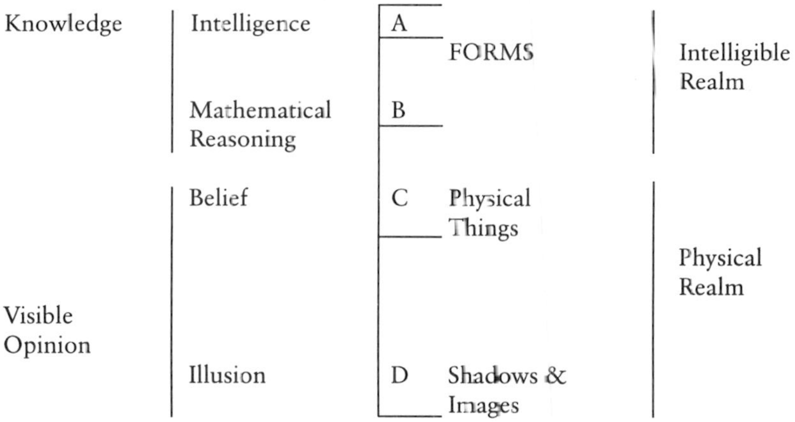

Knowledge	Intelligence	A		Intelligible Realm
			FORMS	
	Mathematical Reasoning	B		
	Belief	C	Physical Things	
				Physical Realm
Visible Opinion				
	Illusion	D	Shadows & Images	

Figure 2.2. Divided-Line Analogy

SOURCE: Adapted with permission of Penguin Books Ltd. from *The Republic* by Plato, translated by Desmond Lee (Penguin Classics, 1935; second revised edition, 1987, p. 310). Copyright © H. D. P. Lee, 1953, 1974, 1987.

become capable of determining the forms that are eternal and un-changing and constitute true knowledge.

Because true knowledge can be discerned only by the intellect, as Plato (1966) argued in the *Meno,* that true knowledge resides within the soul and can be brought to light by astute questioning. To support this claim, he described questioning an uneducated boy who, under the guidance of Socratic reasoning, displayed a remarkable grasp of geometric principles. On the basis of this empirical example, Plato, speaking through the voice of Socrates, stated, "If then there are going to exist within him, both while he is and is not a man, true opinions which can be aroused by questioning and turned into knowledge, may we say that his soul has forever been in a state of knowledge?" (p. 115). Plato made the point that although we know, we do not know that we know. Thus, for Plato, the task of the teacher is to facilitate the student's coming to know what he already knows but does not know that he knows. In this, Plato, in company with Descartes, endorses the rationalist position, which holds that "ideas of reason intrinsic to the mind are the only source of knowledge" (Flew, 1984, p. 109).

Rationalism, as described by Plato and Descartes, is diametrically opposite to empiricism, as first expounded by Locke and Hume. Whereas the rationalists regard necessary truths, theorems, maxims, definitions, and universals as the source of real knowledge, empiricists believe knowledge is derived from experience in that "sense experi-ence is the primary source of our ideas, and hence of knowledge" (Flew, 1984, p. 109). To that extent, rationalism is essentially mathe-matical, whereas empiricism is essentially scientific. However, al-though rationalists and empiricists differ substantially in their claims regarding the source of knowledge, both counter the charges of skepticism, which doubts that anything can be known. It was largely for this reason that Descartes first propounded his now-famous phrase *"cogito ergo sum,"* the meaning of which is that having an awareness of one's thoughts places one's existence beyond doubt.

In this chapter, I argue that knowledge, generally speaking, and nursing knowledge in particular are derived from the interplay between rationalism and empiricism. Or, to put it another way, they are derived from the interplay between philosophical reasoning and science.[2] This interplay is operative in what I am proposing to be four broad levels of knowledge, each of which contributes to the sum total of nursing knowledge. Whereas the first three levels relate to nonpropositional knowledge, the fourth pertains to propositional knowledge only.

Four Levels of Knowledge

The lowest level of knowledge, Level I, includes instinctive, culturally independent behavior (satisfaction of basic physiological needs); subjective knowledge (understanding of one's motivation for action); and affective knowledge (the capacity to empathize and sympathize with others). The criterion by which possession of such knowledge can be evaluated is the extent to which the agent behaves as a rational human being.

Level II rests primarily on the mastery of psychomotor skills, which may range, for example, from bicycle riding to performing sophisticated surgery. The mastery of psychomotor skills constitutes nonpropositional (practical) knowledge, and the criterion by which possession of such knowledge may be evaluated is the level of competence attained in the performance of a particular psychomotor task.

Level III includes culturally dependent knowledge, such as knowledge of English literature, 14th-century poetry, Renaissance art, or the customs and beliefs of other cultures.

Finally, Level IV includes propositional knowledge, which embraces true, justified beliefs acquired by some reliable mechanism. Provision for the acquisition of true, justified beliefs by some reliable mechanism allows for both articulated knowledge and nonarticulated (perceptual) skills[3] to be included within this level of knowledge. Articulated knowledge includes knowledge from such disciplines as science, mathematics, logic, and certain branches of philosophy. Nonarticulated (perceptual) skills include that perceptual knowledge required to become, for example, an expert nurse (in Benner's sense of "expert"; Benner, 1984), an expert surgeon, or even an expert chicken sexer!

These four levels of knowledge are summarized in Table 2.1.

Both nursing and medicine are essentially applied disciplines that depend upon the acquisition of extensive propositional knowledge in conjunction with the mastery of specific psychomotor skills. For

TABLE 2.1 Levels of Knowledge

Level IV	Propositional knowledge: Articulated knowledge and nonarticulated (perceptual) skills
Level III	Nonpropositional knowledge that is culturally dependent (e.g., English literature)
Level II	Nonpropositional (practical) knowledge
Level I	Instinctive, culturally independent behavior; subjective and affective knowledge

example, the surgeon draws upon an extensive knowledge of anatomy and physiology to perform a surgical procedure competently. That is, the surgeon integrates knowledge that pertains to Level IV with knowledge consistent with Level II. Similarly, nursing knowledge is largely a synthesis of articulated and nonarticulated propositional knowledge (that of Level IV) and the nonpropositional knowledge of Level II. The acquisition of nursing knowledge also requires extensive study of the applied sciences along with mastery of relevant psychomotor skills. However, neither surgeons nor nurses would perform their professional duties competently if they were affectively insensitive to the patient's plight. In fact, it is this very point that Benner and Wrubel (1989) stress in *The Primacy of Caring:* It is the art of empathy that makes the difference between the novice and the expert nurse.

To summarize, nursing knowledge incorporates all four levels of knowledge, and mastery of each level is essential for the development of nursing competence. Affective knowledge (Level I) is critical in the delivery of holistic nursing care; practical (psychomotor) knowledge (Level II) is essential to the performance of most nursing tasks; culturally dependent knowledge (Level III) is important in terms of respecting the patient's cultural customs and beliefs; and propositional knowledge, articulated and nonarticulated (Level IV), is vital for the development and formation of a safe practitioner. Keeping in mind these four levels of knowledge, let us now return to the previously noted distinctions between empiricism and rationalism and examine more closely how each of these perspectives is operative in nursing knowledge, as just described.

Empiricism and Rationalism
in Nursing Knowledge

ROLE OF EMPIRICISM

In terms of empiricism, nursing knowledge falls predominantly within the nonarticulated (perceptual) skills domain of Level IV knowledge. The expert nurse relies heavily on perceptual data to form an accurate diagnostic picture of the patient's current health status. He or she needs perceptual propositional knowledge to know, for example, that a particular patient needs more oxygen and not a bedpan. This may be discerned from the color of the patient's skin, the quality of the patient's respirations, and the relationship of these observations to the patient's illness.

As Benner (1984) has been at pains to point out, this level of nursing knowledge is seldom articulated because, over time, the nurse has internalized a rich storehouse of nonarticulated, perceptual propositional knowledge that has been acquired largely from experience. At a subliminal level, the expert nurse has observed a constant conjunction between certain patient states and certain compromised physical outcomes. To this extent, the expert nurse is a true empiricist. In direct accordance with Hume's (1739/1972) view of epistemology, the nurse has derived a profound knowledge of illness causation from a series of simple sense impressions—from the experience of observing a constant conjunction between patient signs and symptoms and subsequent physiological events. The development of this skill equips the expert nurse with highly predictive powers; it is the reliability of these powers that confirms the truth of the nurse's perceptual propositional knowledge.

ROLE OF RATIONALISM

Although nursing entails primarily an observational skill that relies heavily on nonarticulated propositional knowledge (Level IV) consistent with the principles of empiricism, articulated propositional knowledge (Level IV) consistent with the theory of rationalism is also required in nursing practice. Runes (1974) defined *rationalism* as "a theory of philosophy, in which the criterion of truth is not sensory but intellectual and deductive" (p. 263). This definition accords with three increasingly important areas of nursing knowledge: ethics, bioethics, and patient advocacy. As previously noted, Plato (1987) insisted that beauty-in-itself, goodness-in-itself, and justice-in-itself form the basis of true knowledge. Whereas ethics and bioethics are intrinsic to goodness-in-itself, patient advocacy is a constituent of justice-in-itself.

Professional ethics in both medicine and nursing is becoming more and more complex as advances in medical technology become increasingly sophisticated. Not only do advances in medical technology complicate the professional ethics of medicine and nursing, they also give rise to countless bioethical dilemmas. This is especially true in the areas of in vitro fertilization programs, experimentation with human embryos, the sustaining of life of the extremely premature, and organ donation. In my view, bioethical dilemmas are largely responsible for the tension that exists, in some quarters, between the medical and nursing professions. Such tensions are particularly evident in neonatal intensive care units when a nurse does not want to be the person who administers the last dose of morphine, in oncology units when a nurse's desire to facilitate a death with dignity lies at odds with ninth-hour heroic medical interventions, and in intensive care units when professional disputes arise in relation to the prolongation of life by life support systems when the prognosis for the patient is essentially hopeless.

Unfortunately, the capacity to develop sound ethical guidelines through a process of sophisticated moral reasoning is not generally the forte of either nurses or medical practitioners. This situation exists because both professions are intrinsically grounded in empiricism. Thus the transition to analytic reasoning remains relatively foreign. For this reason, achieving a formal understanding of the principles that govern the resolution of bioethical dilemmas has now become an essential ingredient of the educational programs of medicine and nursing. Professional cohesion between medicine and nursing would be greatly enhanced if the ethical and bioethical substance of such programs were taught to medical and nursing students who would be studying it collaboratively.

Yet another source of increasing tension between medicine and nursing in hospitals is patient advocacy. The exercise of the patient advocate role must be tempered with a considerable degree of prudence and insight, joined with well-developed analytic reasoning skills. It could be argued that retreat into "patient advocacy" on the part of nurses, to some extent, parallels a retreat into "paternalism" on the part of physicians, to the mutual irritation of both professional groups! Katz (1986) eloquently pointed out that physicians often take refuge in paternalism as an unconscious means of avoiding the more intellectually and emotionally rigorous path of seeking informed consent. In this sense, paternalism promises unrealistic protection against discerning the true implications of the terrors of illness, whereas patient advocacy promises unrealistic rescue from the terrors of paternalistic physicians. Thus an unsuspecting nurse, not realizing that both roles are equally defensive in their unconscious motivation, is tempted to counterbalance the physician's protective paternalism with professionally immature, misguided maternalism.

The foregoing point is particularly well illustrated in the following pronouncement by Parker (1987), who, following a claim that patient advocacy originally arose out of "mother surrogacy" (pp. 76-77), confidently asserted:

> The nurse has an understanding of both the patient's views [sic] and the doctor's views [sic]. If these are in conflict the nurse has a critical role in acting for the patient to ensure that the patient's hopes and wishes are in fact fully understood by the doctor and that investigations and treatments are *not* initiated unless the patient is fully informed and is prepared to accept the likely outcomes. (p. 81)

This piece of professional enlightenment would be admirable if nurses could be relied upon to understand "both the patient's views and the doctor's views" and to analyze the psychological dynamics of their respective situations accurately. However, I do not believe that nurses are any more generously endowed with this intrinsically insightful capacity than are physicians. It is nothing more than a consummate piece of professional arrogance to assume that "mother" always knows best!

As previously stated, the rationalist tradition adheres to a criterion of truth that is both intellectual and deductive. This means that a sound conceptual framework must form the foundation of both bioethics and patient advocacy if these areas of nursing discourse are to satisfy the rationalist criterion of truth. Katz (1986) pointed out that paternalism, which is inherent in medicine, is essentially defensive and owes its origin to unconscious forces. Also, "mother surrogacy" is thought to have strong unconscious emotional underpinnings that frequently reflect traces of envy (Klein, 1957/1988). Both these motivations violate the requirement that bioethics and patient advocacy be theoretically derived from a process of analytic and deductive reasoning. The task ahead for nursing theorists is, therefore, to produce a sound theoretical base from which bioethics and patient advocacy may develop.

To summarize, before moving ahead, whereas empiricism informs nursing practice, rationalism informs nursing theory, and each tradition has its own criterion of truth. Empiricism relies on the constant conjunction that obtains between a cause and an event, consistent with the Humean criterion of truth. Rationalism, on the other hand, relies upon the laws of logic consistent with the philosophical tradition of argument. Nursing must achieve mastery of both.

Criteria for Identifying
Nursing Knowledge

Thus far, it has been established that nursing knowledge incorporates (a) nonpropositional knowledge that includes empathy, the art of emotional knowing (Holden, 1990a), which is largely affective knowledge; psychomotor skills that constitute practical knowledge; and culturally dependent knowledge; and (b) propositional knowledge that may be of either the articulated or the nonarticulated form (perceptual skills). But by what criteria can the existence of such nursing knowledge be actually identified? In Australia, the Australian Nurse Registering Authorities Conference (ANRAC) identified an impressive set of nursing competencies (ANRAC Nursing Competencies) derived from those enumerated by Benner (1984). These are considered to be the minimum required standards to be met, for the purposes of registration, by a beginning-level practitioner in Australia (Butler et al., 1990, pp. 82-84). The competencies, in abbreviated form, are as follows:

Professional/Ethical Practice

1. Demonstrates a satisfactory knowledge base for safe practice.
2. Functions in accordance with legislation and common law affecting nursing practice.
3. Protects the rights of individuals and groups.
4. Demonstrates accountability for nursing practice.
5. Conducts nursing practice in a way that can be ethically justified.

Reflective Practice

6. Recognises own abilities and level of professional competence.
7. Acts to enhance the professional development of self and others.
8. Recognises the value of research in contributing to developments in nursing and improved standards of care.

Enabling

9. Maintains a physical and psychosocial environment which promotes safety, security and optimal health.
10. Acts to enhance the dignity and integrity of individuals and groups.
11. Assists individuals or groups to make informed decisions.
12. Communicates effectively and documents relevant information.
13. Effectively manages the nursing care of individuals or groups.

Problem Framing and Solving

14. Carries out a comprehensive and accurate nursing assessment of individuals and groups in a variety of settings.
15. Formulates a plan of care in consultation with individuals/groups taking into account the therapeutic regimes of other members of the health care team.
16. Implements planned care.

17. Evaluates progress toward expected outcomes and reviews plans in
accordance with evaluation data.

Teamwork

18. Collaborates with the health care team.[4]

On close examination, it can readily be appreciated that these
competencies embrace each of the four levels of knowledge identified
earlier. For example, the competencies listed under "Professional/
Ethical Practice" embrace propositional knowledge in the articulated
and nonarticulated form (Level IV) as well as nonpropositional knowledge consistent with Level III. The competencies listed under "Reflective Practice" rely heavily on an interplay between propositional
knowledge (Level IV) and nonpropositional (practical) knowledge
(Level II), whereas the competencies included under "Enabling" in-
voke all four levels of knowledge, with particular emphasis on the
empathic skills consistent with Level I and the nonpropositional
knowledge consistent with Level III. The competencies that make up
"Problem Framing and Solving" are intended to embrace nursing
within general hospital and primary health care settings and, once
again, depend on the interplay of propositional and nonpropositional
knowledge (at Levels IV and II, respectively) for their performance.
Finally, "Teamwork" emphasizes collaboration and cooperation both
interprofessionally and intraprofessionally. The exercise of such teamwork indubitably depends upon personal and professional maturity,
which is achieved only through a process of emotional and intellectual
development. Whereas emotional maturity is a key factor in the areas
of affective and subjective knowledge consistent with Level I, intellectual maturity is achieved only through a prolonged educational process in which consistent rigorous demands are made on the person to
acquire propositional and nonpropositional knowledge consistent
with Levels IV and III, respectively. This form of nursing knowledge
is, in fact, most important, for it is politically essential that the
members of the nursing profession demonstrate a willingness actively
to maintain collaborative relationships among themselves and with
other professional members of the health care team.

Conclusion

Because nursing, like medicine, is very much an applied discipline, it has been difficult in the past to define accurately and to identify what comes under the umbrella of nursing knowledge. In an effort to demonstrate that nursing does indeed possess a discrete knowledge base that is unique to the profession, there has been a temptation, on the part of some, to try to manufacture nursing knowledge artificially in an intellectual vacuum. I specifically refer here to the proliferation of nursing models and theories that have done little to enhance the intellectual credibility and respect of nursing. As I have argued elsewhere (Holden, 1990b), these "theories" are little more than prescriptions for action in that they do not satisfy the criteria demanded of a theory in any expected scientific sense or in any expected philosophical sense. Thus nursing models fail to satisfy either the empiricist or the rationalist criteria of knowledge.

In this chapter, I have attempted to demonstrate that nursing knowledge does in fact exist and therefore need not be artificially manufactured. I have argued that *knowledge* can be propositional and nonpropositional, a statement that gives further credence to the claim that nursing is both an art and a science. As an art, nursing rests on the delicate interplay between propositional knowledge (articulated and nonarticulated) and nonpropositional knowledge associated with the mastery of psychomotor skills. As a science, nursing draws heavily on propositional scientific knowledge that is then applied in the practical area. But most important, it is the "expert nurses," with their impressive reservoir of nonarticulated, perceptual propositional knowledge, who transport nursing from a humdrum world of honest toil to the scientific realm of creative caring.

Notes

1. In contemporary philosophical discourse, Plato's position is referred to as Realism, which Aristotle originally countered with Nominalism. Nominalism is a position that argues that universals have no independent existence and exist only insofar as they reside in a given particular. For example, redness is a universal that standardly inheres in

particulars such as fire engines, whiteness standardly inheres in snow, and blueness standardly inheres in the sky. But neither red, white, nor blue assumes an independent existence beyond the particulars in which the universal is vested (Flew, 1984; Runes, 1974).

    2. It is important to note that in philosophy there are two kinds of truths: necessary and contingent. A sentence or proposition that contains a necessary truth is true by virtue of the meaning of the words. For example, take the sentence "All bachelors are unmarried men." Because the meaning of the word *bachelor* is "a man who is not married," the sentence "All bachelors are unmarried men" is necessarily true. Other necessary truths are truths that are essentially mathematical, such as "2 + 3 = 5" or "7 + 3 = 10," or essentially axiomatic, such as "What is, is" and "It is impossible for the same thing to be and not to be." On the other hand, contingent truths require empirical verification to confirm their truth status. For example, take the sentences "The grass is green" and "Today it is raining." To confirm or deny the truth of such sentences, one must look to various aspects of the real (concrete) world.

    3. I owe the distinction drawn between articulated propositional knowledge and nonarticulated (perceptual) skills to Dr. John Burgess, Department of Philosophy, University of Wollongong, New South Wales, Australia.

    4. Reprinted, as abbreviated, with permission of the Australian Nursing Council Inc., from *ANRAC Nursing Competencies Assessment Project: Vol. 1. The Project Report* (pp. 82-84) by the Australian Nurse Registering Authorities Conference. Copyright © 1990 by the Australian Nursing Council Inc.

References

Benner, P. (1984). *From novice to expert: Excellence and power in clinical nursing practice.* New York: Addison-Wesley.

Benner, P., & Wrubel, J. (1989). *The primacy of caring: Stress and coping in health and illness.* New York: Addison-Wesley.

Butler, J., Alavi, C., Bartlett, L., Beasley, W., Fox-Young, S., Kerven, B., Maxwell, G., Sadler, R., & Wilkes, R. (1990). *ANRAC Nursing Competencies Assessment Project: Vol 1. The project report.* Adelaide: Australian Nurse Registering Authorities Conference.

Flew, A. (Ed.). (1984). *A dictionary of philosophy.* London: Pan.

Holden, R. J. (1990a). Empathy: The art of "emotional knowing" in holistic nursing care. *Holistic Nursing Practice, 5,* 70-79.

Holden, R. J. (1990b). Models, muddles and medicine. *International Journal of Nursing Studies, 27,* 223-234.

Hume, D. (1972). *A treatise of human nature, Book I.* London: Fontana. (Original work published 1739)

Katz, J. (1986). *The silent world of doctor and patient.* New York: Free Press.

Klein, M. (1988). Envy and gratitude. In M. Klein, *Envy and gratitude and other works: 1946-1963* (pp. 176-235). London: Virago. (Original work published 1957)

Parker, J. (1987). The nurse as patients' advocate. In J. Hudson (Ed.), *Proceedings of the Centre for Human Bioethics Conference on the Role of the Nurse: Doctors' Handmaiden, Patients' Advocate or What?* (pp. 85-91). Clayton, Australia: Monash University, Monash Centre for Human Bioethics.

Plato. (1966). *Meno.* In R. E. Allen (Ed.) & W. K. C. Guthrie (Trans.), *Greek philosophy: Thales to Aristotle* (pp. 97-128). New York: Free Press.

Plato. (1987). *The Republic* (2nd ed., D. Lee, Trans.). Harmondsworth: Penguin.

Runes, D. D. (Ed.). (1974). *Dictionary of philosophy.* Totowa, NJ: Littlefield, Adams.

CHAPTER 3

Nursing Art and Prescriptive Truths

JOY L. JOHNSON

The proper place of prescriptive theory within the nursing discipline has been vigorously debated. This debate became most heated in the 1970s, when authors such as Beckstrand (1978a, 1978b, 1980); Dickoff, James, and Wiedenbach (1968a, 1968b); Jacox (1974); and Walker (1971) entered into a dialogue about what came to be known as "practice theory." These authors ought to be commended for their pioneering philosophical efforts. Rather than simply putting forth their own points of view, they joined issue on what is perhaps one of nursing's most controversial topics.

Although the debate regarding the proper place of practice theory in nursing diminished in intensity in the 1980s, on occasion, nursing scholars take up the gauntlet and continue to address this important issue. Unfortunately, rather than bringing us closer to an understanding of the proper place of practice theory, much of the debate has obfuscated rather than clarified the issues. This is, in part, because the example of Beckstrand, Dickoff et al., Jacox, and Walker is not emulated. Nurses have not joined issue in relation to this topic, and consequently it is difficult to determine if genuine disagreement about the role of practice theory persists.

The topic of prescriptive truth, which is addressed in this chapter, is highly related to the topic of practice theory. Indeed, the proper place of prescriptions has often been the point of contention in debates about practice theory. The purpose of this chapter is twofold. First, I attempt to clarify what has often been an extremely confusing topic of discussion by outlining three contrary positions. Second, I critically examine those positions with a view to determining which is the most sound.

Illustrating the importance of providing clear definitions in the philosophical enterprise, Maritain (1979) reminded us that "before sewing one must cut" (p. 76). Similarly, a philosopher in search of an answer to a complex question must begin with sharp distinctions if a coherent argument is to be made. Accordingly, I will begin by defining some key terms and setting out the assumptions upon which my arguments rest.

Definitions

The claim is often made that nursing is an art. Unfortunately, what is meant by the term *nursing art* remains obscure. In light of the indeterminacy of the term, a fairly broad definition will be used in this chapter. Art, it is generally agreed, is concerned with making a thing well. For example, the art of painting is what enables the painter to make a beautiful painting, and the art of shoemaking is what enables the shoemaker to make excellent shoes. Nursing art, then, is what enables a person to nurse in an excellent manner.

But what kind of an art is nursing art? All art is productive in that the operations of art terminate in the production of an effect (Adler, 1937). But the kinds of changes that art brings about differ significantly from one kind of art to another. Adler (1937) contended that kinds of art can be distinguished on the basis of the kind of change brought about. He asserted that practical arts involve accidental change in a substance, whereas productive arts bring about a change that has been individually created through a unique composition of accidental and substantial changes. Accordingly, productive arts, such as shipbuilding and sculpting, work by operating on nature and by imposing a form on the materials being used. In contrast, the practical arts, such as teaching and medicine, effect changes that might occur without the intervention of the artist in that the changes are due to active principles in the natural order. Rather than operating *on* nature, the practical artist works by "cooperating with nature" (Adler, 1937, p. 433). It would seem that nursing art is not a productive art but rather a practical art in that the effects that nurses attempt to bring about, such as changes in health, are natural changes. Using this distinction, *nursing art* can be defined as a practical art that perfects a nurse's practice.

Truth is a content of knowledge or a proposition to which truth belongs. When we think of truth, we often think of knowledge that is certain, indubitable, and incorrigible. However, little of human knowledge meets this exacting definition. Indeed, it would seem that certainty is left to knowledge of self-evident truths or axioms, such as the claim that a triangle has no diagonals, and the conclusions rigorously developed from such self-evident truths. I use the term *truth* not in this strong sense but rather to designate propositions that are testable by reference to evidence, subject to rational criticism, corrigible and rectifiable, or falsifiable (Adler, 1965). Though not meeting the exacting criterion of certainty, this notion of probable truth is set apart from personal opinion and knowledge of our personal experiences.

We can distinguish further between two kinds of truth: speculative and prescriptive. Whereas speculative truth refers to that which is the case, prescriptive truth deals specifically with the realm of action, or what ought to be done. The object of prescriptive truth is not truth alone, but a performable good. Prescriptive truths can be thought of as rules or directives that guide action. This is not to say that prescriptive and speculative truths are unrelated; prescriptive truths presuppose speculative truths. Maritain (1959) claimed that knowledge of prescriptions is based on theoretical, speculative, and explanatory knowledge of things that need to be explained as well as things that need to be done. One cannot develop sound principles to guide action unless one first possesses knowledge about the end that is to be achieved and the factors that may influence achievement of that end. Thus, for example, one must possess speculative knowledge regarding the nature of a bridge and the factors that operate on the structure of a bridge, such as weather, gravity, and traffic load, before one can create sound prescriptions for bridge making. Unlike speculative truths, prescriptive truths directly regulate practice and bear on particular operations.

The ancient philosophers made a further distinction between two kinds of prescriptive truths. Aristotle (1941) contended that each human activity is directed toward some good and on this basis argued that "the reasoned state of capacity to act is different from the reasoned state of capacity to make" (pp. 1025, 1140a 4-5). Prescriptions that deal with making things and with achieving desired effects or results can be referred to as *artistic prescriptive truths*. Artistic prescriptive truths are directed toward the good of a particular work. A second kind of prescriptive truth has to do with individual conduct or doing and is referred to as *moral prescriptive truth*. Moral prescriptive truths serve, not the good of a particular work, but the good of human beings. More will be said about these two kinds of prescriptive truths later. When I use the term *prescriptive truth* in this chapter, I am referring to both artistic and moral prescriptions unless otherwise stated. Furthermore, the term *prescriptive truth* will be used to refer to nursing prescriptive truths—that is, prescriptions about how one ought to nurse versus how one ought to paint, fix a car, or build a bridge.

Assumptions

The arguments presented in this chapter rest on two related assumptions. First, I am assuming a realistic epistemology. This position holds that reality exists external to us and that it is possible to obtain probable truths about reality. Second, I am assuming that philosophy is not a matter of mere opinion and that we can obtain philosophic truths by reflecting on and discursively analyzing our commonsense knowledge (what we know by virtue of our common sense operating on our common experience; Adler, 1993).

Having provided some key definitions and outlined the major assumptions of my argument, I now turn to the topic of discussion. The specific question I propose to address is "What is the relationship between prescriptive truth and nursing art?" I plan to proceed by considering three contrary positions. One position holds that there is no relationship between the possession of prescriptive truth and nursing art. A second holds that the possession of prescriptive truth is a necessary and sufficient condition for nursing art. A third holds that the possession of prescriptive truth is a necessary but not sufficient condition for nursing art. Each of these positions will be considered in turn.

Prescriptive Truth and Nursing Art:
Three Positions

NO RELATIONSHIP BETWEEN
PRESCRIPTIVE TRUTH AND NURSING ART

Those who hold that there is no relationship between prescriptive truth and nursing art argue that a nurse can be artful without possessing prescriptive nursing truths. Two central claims are employed in defense of this position. First, it is contended that there is no such thing as prescriptive truth and that because of this there is no relationship between prescriptive truth and nursing art. According to this view, there is no basis for making valid or truthful prescriptive claims; prescriptive truth, therefore, is believed to be no more than personal value judgment about what is desirable.

We are correctly reminded by those who hold this position of the perils of the naturalistic fallacy: namely, that a prescriptive conclusion cannot be validly derived from premises that are entirely descriptive. In other words, merely because something is the case does not necessarily mean that it ought to be the case. Is this, then, the fatal blow to prescriptive truth, or are there means by which we can affirm the truth of prescriptive conclusions? The solution to the problem can be located in the work of Aristotle (1941), who suggested that reasoning, in the form of a practical syllogism, can be used to establish prescriptive truth. In a practical syllogism, the major premise must be a prescriptive truth about what ought to be desired or done; the accompanying minor premise must be a descriptive truth about a matter of fact relevant to what ought to be desired or done. The conclusion reached by reasoning from the major and minor premises is a further prescriptive truth. Let me provide two examples of a practical syllogism.

A *moral* prescriptive truth might be reached in the following manner. The major premise is "Nurses ought to treat patients with respect." (I doubt that anyone would challenge this claim.) The minor premise is descriptive: "Respect for another is demonstrated by introducing oneself to the patient." The conclusion reached by this reasoning takes the form "Nurses ought to introduce themselves to their patients." This prescription is moral because it is aimed at serving the good of human beings and not that of a particular work in nursing per se.

A second example outlines how *artistic* prescriptions might be deduced. The major premise takes the form "The introduction of bacteria ought to be avoided when dressing surgical wounds." The minor premise takes the form "The use of sterile technique when dressing surgical wounds prevents the introduction of bacteria." The conclusion that follows from these premises is "Sterile technique ought to be used when dressing surgical wounds." This conclusion is an artistic prescriptive truth that pertains to making a good dressing. Although simplistic, these syllogisms demonstrate how prescriptive truths can be validly developed.

It might be argued that the reasoning used in these syllogisms is somewhat circular in that we still must deal with the question of how the major premises are derived. Basing his position on the work of Aristotle, Adler (1981) correctly claimed that the only self-evident moral prescription is that we ought to desire what is really good for us. This principle is self-evident because it is obvious that no one would desire what was bad for him or her. This self-evident principle can serve as the major premise of the initial practical syllogism. However, the identification of this axiom offers only a partial solution to the problem of circularity; we still are left to determine what is really good for us.

The work of Wallace (1984) offers a solution to the problem of circularity in developing practical syllogisms. He contended that speculative understanding of human nature provides the necessary background for the study of activity that is perfective of the individual. In other words, an understanding of the nature of human beings and of inherent human needs can provide the basis for the development of prescriptions for human behavior. The prescriptive premises used in practical syllogisms can be determined by understanding that what is really good is what meets a human need. Thus prescriptive truths are grounded in an objective standard: human nature.

Just as moral prescriptive premises can be derived from understanding human nature, the premises used in syllogistic reasoning about artistic nursing prescriptions can be determined by understanding the nature of nursing practice. Maritain (1979) pointed out that a splendid house without a doorway is not an example of good architecture. The architect who designs such a house does not understand the nature of houses. An understanding of the nature of houses provides the basis for sound prescriptions for the art of house design. Similarly, if we understand the nature of nursing practice and if human health is determined to be the proper goal or end of nursing, prescriptive nursing truths will be grounded in an understanding of how the nurse cooperates with nature to "make" health in the human being. Further, the better we understand the nature of human health, the better we will understand the means by which we can intervene to help an individual achieve health. Rather than resting on what an individual desires (i.e., what I want or what you want), prescriptive truth is grounded in an understanding of human nature and what humans naturally need, in the case of moral prescriptions, or what the work requires, in the case of artistic prescriptions.

A second point made in attempts to refute the connection between prescriptive truths and nursing art is the claim that it is inappropriate to use prescriptions when dealing with autonomous and free individuals. This claim is based on the assumption that individuals are entirely autonomous and that the artful nurse must respect the choices of each patient. Support for this claim is found in the works of nursing scholars such as Allen (1985), Gadow (1980), Newman (1986), and Parse (1981). Parse, for example, contended that nursing art must be grounded in the patient's understanding of the situation and that nursing practice is "unencumbered by prescriptive rules" (p. 81). Similarly, Allen claimed that the use of means-end reasoning leads to an objectification of the patient. Though Allen acknowledged that such reasoning may be necessary for what he termed "technical decisions," such as those necessitated by medical emergencies, he claimed that it is inappropriate to use such an approach in the indeterminate client situation in that it disregards the individuality of the client.

We have a great deal to sort out about the proper place of client autonomy in nursing practice. True autonomy, it would seem, can be possessed only by individuals who lead completely solitary lives; yet human beings live in relation to one another. Practices such as nursing seem to have no place in a social climate that values autonomy above all else. As nurses, we must ask, "Are there principles other than autonomy that are applicable to human beings?" Dreher (1982) offered some alternative principles. She suggested that principles regarding cleanliness, appropriate clothing, and good nutrition are not simply matters of cultural mores or value judgments, but health principles that are equally applicable to all human beings.

Though perhaps not wholly autonomous, individuals do have the right to make decisions about their lives. However, it cannot be concluded that a nurse's use of prescriptive truths, or means-ends reasoning, necessarily violates the individual's right to make choices or designates individuals as objects. The claim that an artful nurse requires prescriptive truths does not mean that he or she blindly applies such truths to the individual case without consideration of the patient's values and desires.

It is instructive to consider how the artful nurse would operate in the absence of prescriptive truths. Without prescriptive truths, the nurse is left to base his or her decisions either on personal opinion, wants, or desires or on the opinion, wants, or desires of the patient. What occurs when the nurse bases decisions on the desires of the patient? Because they often lack the necessary knowledge and skill, patients generally rely on professional nurses to work with them to bring about changes in their health status. To do solely as a patient wishes or desires might not be in the patient's best interest. For example, consider a patient who, for whatever reason, asks the nurse not to use sterile technique when changing his or her dressing. Is it the nurse's duty to respect this wish or to help the patient to understand the need for sterile technique? A patient who makes decisions based on ignorance is not truly making an informed decision.

Let us consider the alternative of basing decisions on the nurse's personal opinion. The problem with this approach is that it affirms the power of the individual nurse to make decisions. Anyone who has worked with first-year student nurses or with nurses who are religious zealots can readily appreciate the limitations of this approach. Both of these groups of individuals possess many opinions; however, we do not encourage them to base their practices on their opinions.

In ancient times, the empiric in medicine was one who lacked the art of healing because, lacking the relevant sciences, he worked by trial and error rather than in the light of fixed rules (Adler, 1937). Similarly, without an arsenal of prescriptive truths, nurses will be left to flounder as they attempt to determine how to proceed and will face insurmountable obstacles as they attempt to perfect their practices. Maritain (1962) contended that without the rational application of prescriptive truths, the fine arts are nothing more than "sensual slush" (p. 38). I believe the same conclusion may be drawn for nursing art.

Finally, it should be pointed out that no matter how determined we may be to avoid prescriptive truths, when we deal with the realm of action, they seem to be present either implicitly or explicitly. For example, Gadow's (1980) claim that "self-determination ought not to be infringed upon" is a prescription (p. 85). The irony is that in making what might be construed to be an argument against the use of prescriptions, Gadow is forced to cite a proposition that is prescriptive. As members of a learned profession, it is important that we make explicit the assumptions on which we think and act so that they may be duly considered and, as necessary, amended. Accordingly, it is important that nurses explicitly acknowledge that prescriptive truths are important for artful nursing and that these truths should be explicitly stated and fully considered. The alternative is to use an implicit network of prescriptive truths that are difficult to analyze and understand.

PRESCRIPTIVE TRUTHS ARE NECESSARY
AND SUFFICIENT FOR NURSING ART

A second position taken on the question of the relationship between prescriptive truth and nursing art holds that the possession of prescriptive truth is both a necessary and a sufficient condition for nursing art. According to this position, practical arts, such as nursing, are entirely determined by the application of prescriptive rules. Accordingly, there is identity between the possession of prescriptive truth and nursing art. Much like the rules of a game, prescriptive truths are viewed as a self-complete sort of knowledge that guides action. Thus, if one thoroughly knows the rules, one can effectively practice nursing. This position is supported by nursing scholars such as Mallick (1981), who criticized the vague principles used to gather assessment information, contending that rigorous nursing practice ideally involves the use of preestablished and rigorously tested procedures. Using a similar line of argument, Beckstrand (1978a, 1978b) contended that artful nursing practice involves determining the relevant conditions that exist in a patient's situation and logically determining the ethical and scientific knowledge that should be applied to the problems identified.

Drawing on the work of Schön (1983), several nursing scholars have referred to the practice of rationally applying interventions to practice as "technical rationality." Schön used this term to refer to the approach in which decisions are made by selecting and simply applying the best of available means to an identified problem. Schön aptly pointed out that the problem with this approach is that clinical situations are often very complex, uncertain, and unstable and that prescriptive truths cannot be readily applied to the identified problem by the artful practitioner.

The knowledge required for resolving the problems of nursing practice clearly involves more than prescriptive truths. It seems that no matter how complete a list of prescriptive truths may be, it can never be sufficient for artful nursing. In other words, to realize their visions, nurse artists must possess prescriptive truths and not be possessed by them. Plainly, as being an artful cook involves more than following a recipe, artful nursing involves more than merely following

a set of prescriptions. Tanner's (1988) observation that she has encountered students who can write elegant nursing care plans but
cannot respond to rapidly changing situations attests to the claim that
knowing a set of prescriptive rules is not enough for artful nursing.

PRESCRIPTIVE TRUTHS ARE NECESSARY
BUT NOT SUFFICIENT FOR NURSING ART

A third position taken in relation to the question "What is the
relationship between prescriptive truth and nursing art?" is that
prescriptive truths are a necessary but *not* a sufficient condition for
artful nursing practice. I contend that this third position provides the
most sound answer to the question posed.

Why are prescriptive truths necessary for nursing art? To answer
this question, let us consider whether there are any alternatives. As
discussed earlier, two alternatives to basing one's practice on prescriptive truths are to base it on either the nurse's or the patient's personal
opinions. A third alternative that has not yet been considered is to base
nursing art on speculative nursing science. It is this approach that
caused Rogers (1964) to observe, "The art of nursing develops only
as it incorporates more and more science unto itself" (p. 32). The
difficulty with this alternative is that it is not clear how speculative
scientific findings can be translated into artful nursing. For example,
how can a scientific proposition of the form "Continuous tube feeding,
rather than bolus feeding, decreases the incidence of diarrhea" be used
to perfect a nurse's practice? Only when this proposition is translated
into a guide for effective action can the knowledge be used. The
nurse's use of such knowledge is inevitably directed by such beliefs as
"Nurses ought to prevent diarrhea." Again, is it not preferable to make
these prescriptions explicit? The prescriptive truths that guide nursing
practice are partially derived from scientific principles. It is for this
reason that every art can be called a science. What is formulated
prescriptively as the rules of art can also be formulated declaratively
as scientific principles (Adler, 1937).

Prescriptive truths are necessary for nursing art because they ground
decision making. Artful nurses can employ prescriptive truths to guide
their actions and to evaluate outcomes. Explicitly stated and sharable,

prescriptive truths are amenable to critique, modification, and correction. Nursing art is highly contingent on having the best possible directives for practice. The development of prescriptions is likely to be facilitated if they are shared. Thus it is inadvisable for practitioners to be left to translate speculative scientific findings into practice independently.

My comments regarding the necessity of prescriptive truths have been limited, thus far, to a discussion of artistic prescriptions. One might ask if the possession of moral prescriptive truths is also required for artful nursing. Some might argue that moral prescriptive truths are not required in that nursing art deals with the realm of making, not the realm of doing. Accordingly, art is viewed as autonomous in its own sphere in that only art determines the means to be used in accomplishing its particular end. I am not convinced of the correctness of this answer. I am inclined to agree with Curtin (1979), who described nursing as a moral art. Unlike fine artists, such as painters and poets, nurses deal directly with human lives as they "make" their art. The artistic decisions nurses make have direct consequences for other lives. For this reason, I am inclined to conclude that nurses cannot perfect their practice unless they possess moral as well as artistic prescriptions.

Why are prescriptive truths not sufficient? As previously discussed, artful nursing involves more than rigidly following a set of prescriptions. Nurses deal with unique human beings and unique circumstances. What may seem to be a most obvious prescription, such as "Nurses ought to use sterile technique when dressing surgical wounds," must at times be modified or entirely disregarded. For example, in certain life-threatening situations, it may be inappropriate to don sterile gloves. Similarly, the prescription that "nurses ought to introduce themselves to their patients" must be interpreted by the nurse and applied appropriately. If a patient is observed to be in deep conversation with family members, it may be inappropriate for the nurse to introduce himself- or herself. Rules alone, no matter how explicit, will never be sufficient for artful nursing. In addition to prescriptive truths, the artful nurse must possess "artistic nursing prudence." In the same way that Adler (1937) defined *artistic prudence,* artistic nursing prudence is what enables the nurse to choose wisely and well about how nursing prescriptive truths ought to be applied in the particular case. Dickoff et al. (1968b) recognized the limitations of rules and argued that the artful nurse must possess the capacity "to consult all salient features in the particular situation and make adjustments of a more routine activity in the light of any idiosyncratic (that is, nonroutine) characteristics" (p. 422).

Besides artistic prudence, are there other conditions that complement prescriptive truths and contribute to the perfection of nursing practice? I will conclude by suggesting some additional conditions that may be necessary for nursing art. These suggestions are drawn primarily from the work of Maritain (1960, 1962, 1979). One possible condition is that the nurse possess a productive idea of what he or she wants to accomplish. Having a creative idea does not make superfluous the possession of prescriptive truths. On the contrary, it demands that the nurse use these truths as necessary instruments. As such, prescriptive truths are used by the artful nurse as instruments of creative intuition. Without this creative intuition, the nurse may perform individual tasks correctly but in the end produce nothing. Nurses must know what they hope to achieve with patients if they are to ensure that their actions are beneficial. It is this creative intuition that is the driving force behind nursing actions. Without this vision, there is no guarantee that anything of use will be accomplished.

Another possible condition for artful nursing is that the nurse possess know-how. Maritain (1979) claimed that art is a virtue of the practical intellect and that manual skill in making (i.e., manual dexterity) is a material, extrinsic condition of art. It is this position that led Maritain to conclude that art is never mistaken. He argued that the artist who possesses the virtue of art and a trembling hand produces an imperfect work but retains a faultless virtue. It is for this reason that manual skill is not part of art itself but a material and extrinsic condition of it. Nurses must possess the skill that enables them to handle equipment and to communicate effectively if they are to realize their artistic visions.

A third possible condition is that the nurse artist possess a love of the thing to be made. Maritain (1962) claimed that undeviating love is the supreme rule of art. Nurses' passion for their work helps to ensure that the work is accomplished in an excellent manner. It is the love of the work that engenders pride of craftsmanship and "the pleasure felt in the very doing" (Dickoff et al., 1968b, p. 433). Like all artists (Maritain, 1979), nurse artists are not necessarily in love with what they are doing but rather with what they are doing it for. It is the love of the work that causes a nurse to pay attention to detail and to remain vigilant despite difficult circumstances. Lanara (1981) contended that a nurse requires a certain heroism to be true to the work.

A final suggestion is that artful nursing requires the possession of habitus. Habitus, Maritain (1962) pointed out, is a stable disposition to act in a certain way that is acquired through exercise and use. Knowledge of prescriptive truths relevant to nursing practice is not sufficient. These truths must not simply be understood but must be possessed by the nurse artist as habits of proceeding in definite and fixed ways for the accomplishment of the work. Maritain claimed that even if one were to "plaster the perfect theoretical knowledge of all the rules of an art onto an energetic laureate who works fifteen hours a day but in whom habitus is not sprouting, . . . [one would] never make an artist of him" (p. 40). The rules of art must not simply be known by the artist but must be possessed in such a way that he or she seemingly proceeds in a spontaneous and intuitive manner.

In conclusion, the possession of prescriptive truths is a necessary but not sufficient condition for nursing art. Other possible conditions necessary for nursing art include the possession of creative intuition, manual skill, love of the work, and habitus. To draw the conclusion that prescriptive truths are not necessary condemns nursing art to be based on personal opinion; to say that they are necessary and sufficient implies that nursing art must be based on an approach that rigidly applies specified rules. It cannot be concluded that either of these alternatives will contribute to the perfection of nursing practice.

References

Adler, M. J. (1937). *Art and prudence: A study in practical philosophy.* New York: Longmans, Green.
Adler, M. J. (1965). *The conditions of philosophy: Its checkered past, its present disorder, and its future promise.* New York: Atheneum.
Adler, M. J. (1981). *Six great ideas.* New York: Collier.

50   KINDS OF TRUTH IN NURSING INQUIRY

Adler, M. J. (1993). *The four dimensions of philosophy: Metaphysical, moral, objective, categorical.* New York: Macmillan.

Allen, D. (1985). Nursing research and social control: Alternative models of science that emphasize understanding and emancipation. *Image, 17*(2), 58-64.

Aristotle. (1941). Nichomachean ethics (W. D. Ross, Trans.). In R. McKeon (Ed.), *The basic works of Aristotle* (pp. 927-1112). New York: Random House.

Beckstrand, J. (1978a). The notion of a practice theory and the relationship of scientific and ethical knowledge to practice. *Research in Nursing and Health, 1,* 131-136.

Beckstrand, J. (1978b). The need for a practice theory as indicated by the knowledge used in the conduct of practice. *Research in Nursing and Health, 1,* 175-179.

Beckstrand, J. (1980). A critique of several conceptions of practice theory in nursing. *Research in Nursing and Health, 3,* 69-79.

Curtin, L. (1979). The nurse as advocate: A philosophical foundation for nursing. *Advances in Nursing Science, 1*(3), 1-10.

Dickoff, J., James, P., & Wiedenbach, E. (1968a). Theory in a practice discipline, Part I: Practice oriented theory. *Nursing Research, 17,* 415-435.

Dickoff, J., James, P., & Wiedenbach, E. (1968b). Theory in a practice discipline, Part II: Practice oriented research. *Nursing Research, 17,* 545-554.

Dreher, M. C. (1982). The conflict of conservatism in public health nursing education. *Nursing Outlook, 30,* 504-509.

Gadow, S. (1980). Existential advocacy: Philosophical foundation of nursing. In S. F. Spicker & S. Gadow (Eds.), *Nursing images and ideals: Opening dialogue with the humanities* (pp. 79-101). New York: Springer.

Jacox, A. K. (1974). Theory construction in nursing: An overview. *Nursing Research, 23,* 4-13.

Lanara, V. A. (1981). *Heroism as a nursing value: A philosophical perspective.* Athens: Sisterhood Evniki.

Mallick, M. J. (1981). Patient assessment—based on data, not intuition. *Nursing Outlook, 29,* 600-605.

Maritain, J. (1959). *The degrees of knowledge* (G. B. Phelan, Trans.). London: Geoffrey Bles.

Maritain, J. (1960). *The responsibility of the artist.* New York: Scribner.

Maritain, J. (1962). *Art and scholasticism* (J. W. Evans, Trans.). New York: Scribner.

Maritain, J. (1979). Art as a virtue of the practical intellect. In M. Weitz (Ed.), *Problems in aesthetics* (pp. 76-92). London: Macmillan.

Newman, M. A. (1986). *Health as expanding consciousness.* St. Louis: C. V. Mosby.

Parse, R. R. (1981). *Man-living-health: A theory of nursing.* New York: John Wiley.

Rogers, M. E. (1964). *Reveille in nursing.* Philadelphia: F. A. Davis.

Schön, D. A. (1983). *The reflective practitioner: How professionals think in action.* New York: Basic Books.

Tanner, C. (1988). Curriculum revolution: The practice mandate. In National League for Nursing (Ed.), *Curriculum revolution: Mandate for change* (pp. 201-216). New York: National League for Nursing.

Walker, L. O. (1971). Toward a clearer understanding of the concept of nursing theory. *Nursing Research, 20,* 428-435.

Wallace, W. A. (1984). The intelligibility of nature: A neo-Aristotelian view. *Review of Metaphysics, 38,* 33-56.

PART II

Measures of Truth in Nursing Inquiry

In our everyday world, when we claim that we "know" something, it is not unusual to be asked how we know that our claim is true. The more serious the matter, the more we are apt to be asked, and should be asked, for the evidence and/or reasons supportive of our claim. Implicitly, we are being asked what measures of truth lie behind our claim. In nursing research, it is no different.

When nurse researchers assert that they have developed a nursing theory that ought to be applied in nursing practice, practicing nurses ought to ask for the basis of the claim and evaluate that basis before acting. The possibility of carrying out this evaluation, however, is dependent on appropriate measures of truth having been identified. Lives may depend on whether, and how, this evaluation is carried out.

What measures of truth, then, are appropriate in nursing inquiry? Keeping in mind that there are as many measures of truth as there are kinds of truth, this question may be answered, in part, by identifying the kinds of truth that are appropriate to nursing practice. We say *in part* because, before we can determine what kinds of truth are or are not appropriate to nursing practice, we must have a criterion measure against which that differentiation can be made. Further, not all kinds of truth appropriate to nursing practice may be amenable to study in nursing inquiry. To sort out which kinds of truth are or are not amenable to such study, we require, once again, a criterion measure against which that determination can be made.

The importance of identifying appropriate criterion measures of truth in nursing inquiry cannot be overstated. We cannot proceed in our inquiry without them. To attempt to do so is foolhardy, not to mention a waste of precious resources. There is an increasing tendency, of late, for objective measures of truth, traditionally used in nursing inquiry, to be replaced by subjective measures thought to be more appropriate for various reasons. The consequences of this trend for the development of nursing's body of knowledge have yet to become evident. Measures of truth reflective of this new trend can be found implicit in many of the essays included in Part II of this volume.

Measures of truth, as they appear in the first three essays, are based on a conception of humans as continually interacting with, and as coextensive with, their environment. Within this conception, Rew, in Chapter 4, focuses on the individual as a measure of truth in nursing inquiry; Laffrey, in Chapter 5, emphasizes the role of context in terms of community and culture as measures in the attainment of truths in nursing; and Penticuff, in Chapter 6, considers reality, viewed in the context of traditions, as a measure of truth. In the last two chapters of this section, various conceptions of the nature of nursing are examined, using different measures of truth. Bishop, in Chapter 7, uses three essential characteristics of nursing as implicit measures: nursing as a practice, the moral sense of nursing, and nursing as a practice of caring. In Chapter 8, Schlotfeldt uses common sense as yet another measure.

Guiding Questions:
Making up Your Own Mind

Can diverse measures of truth in nursing inquiry come into conflict? If so, by what means, if any, can the conflict(s) be resolved?

Is it necessary to have agreed-upon measures of truth in nursing inquiry?

If reality does not exist independent of the mind, is agreement on measures of truth in nursing inquiry possible?

If truth is a subjective matter only, is a measure of truth necessary?

How might subjective measures of truth arise out of rank skepticism?

If nursing focuses exclusively on objective measures of truth, can its practice requirements be met?

If, in fact, nursing is experiencing an "epistemological crisis," to what degree can that be attributed to the confusion concerning what constitutes an appropriate measure of nursing truth?

How would measures of truth differ if the individual is regarded as coextensive with the environment as opposed to not being coextensive with it?

Under what condition(s) ought one measure of truth in nursing inquiry be replaced with another?

Can common sense and history serve as measures of truth in the advancement of nursing knowledge?

CHAPTER 4

The Individual as a
Measure of Truth
in Nursing Inquiry

LYNN REW

There is something fascinating about the silver-white metallic element of mercury. Mercury has been known to human beings for well over 2,000 years. It has been used for myriad purposes, ranging from the production of cosmetics to that of medicines and from symbolism in religious ceremonies to indication of small temperature changes in scientific instruments. Mercury melts at a temperature of –38 degrees Fahrenheit and boils at a temperature well over 600 degrees Fahrenheit. It is more than 13 times heavier than water and is usually found in its raw form in combination with sulphur in the red mineral cinnabar.

As a child, I first encountered the substance when I accidentally broke a thermometer. As the silvery-white liquid spread over the tabletop, I tried in vain to soak it up with a napkin, only to discover that it either broke apart, forming several little droplets from one large drop, or formed a puddle as several little droplets skittered across the table to pair up with other droplets. Despite my best efforts to be organized, responsible, and intentional in my behavior, I could not soak up the mess I had made.

Since that first experience with mercury, I have learned many truths about this remarkable natural element that have been established through systematic inquiry based on empirical observations. In my attempt to inform you about the physical properties of mercury, I identified some of these established truths about the element. Then, rather than telling you about the scientific phenomenon of surface tension that explains why the mercury from my broken thermometer was not soaked up by the cloth napkin, I described instead my direct encounter with its peculiar characteristics. Unless I am very mistaken, in this description you continued to have glimpses of the truth about mercury.

It is apparent that we humans are curious creatures with a consciousness that allows us to ask all kinds of questions about things such as mercury in our enchanting environments. The intimate relationship between human beings and their environments has traditionally been of interest to nurses. For example, Florence Nightingale (1859/1946), in *Notes on Nursing,* asserted that every woman, at some time in her life, would have to take charge of another person's health. To do that, she thought that a woman would need to have what she referred to as "sanitary knowledge, or the knowledge of nursing," which would be apparent in the "proper use of fresh air, light, warmth, cleanliness, quiet, and the proper selection and administration of diet—all at the least expense of vital power to the patient" (p. 6).

A century later, Virginia Henderson (1966) identified 14 needs of nursing clients, including physical needs such as breathing normally and eating adequately, safety needs such as avoiding environmental hazards, esteem needs such as expressing emotions and needs to others, and self-actualization needs such as learning and developing oneself fully. Her definition of nursing was:

The unique function of the nurse is to assist the individual, sick or well, in the performance of those activities contributing to health or recovery (or to a peaceful death) that he would perform unaided if he had the necessary strength, will, or knowledge. It is likewise her function to help the individual gain independence as rapidly as possible. (p. 4)

Nursing Inquiry and Knowledge

Nursing inquiry is the process of posing and answering questions of interest to the discipline for the purpose of discovering and/or creating truths. Systematic nursing inquiry enables us to understand the phenomena around which the knowledge base of the discipline is organized. It is my thesis that truth in nursing evolves, as a whole over time, through the dynamic relationship between human beings and their environments. A truth in nursing, I submit, is the unity of life. To build the body of nursing knowledge, we must conceive of the human being as an individual, as part of a community and culture, and as part of history and the evolution of consciousness as a repository of nursing truth.

Nursing knowledge includes conceptualizations of the individual person or human being. At this point in our evolution of consciousness, in many of our efforts to study systematically and to understand human phenomena, we must of necessity conceptualize the individual human being using a static or linear model. Implicitly, none of us believes that these conceptualizations, even those that are abstract and multidimensional, adequately reflect the complexity and diversity of what is real and true about the individual. These conceptualizations must not be taken to mean that in the discipline we view the individual as a static object about which "the truth" can be discovered once and for all.

The Individual as a Repository of Truth

In the past century and a half of formal development of the discipline, those of us engaged in systematic nursing inquiry have grappled with philosophies of science and art, abstract and grounded theories, and the matter of the ultimate purpose of our quest for truths in nursing. We have engaged in extensive discourse about our values and beliefs, the boundaries and the phenomena of concern to us, and the methods best suited to answering our questions. We have sought answers to questions at first based primarily on a philosophy of logical positivism and empiricism and more recently based on philosophies such as organicism and historicism (Meleis, 1991). A question of paramount importance to nursing inquiry is "What are valid sources of truth in nursing?"

Nurses and their clients are messengers of truth in nursing. That is, as human beings, both nurse and client carry truths about their individual development embodied physically, expressed psychologically through their temperaments, and enacted socially in their external behaviors. Our personal histories include those genetic indicators that determine who we are, each cell of our individual bodies reflecting the pattern of our uniqueness. Our personal stories or narratives are composites of experience and ways of thinking and knowing that represent the truth of who we are. These personal narratives have been influenced and shaped by our interactions with family, society, and the universe at large. As individuals, we each express a distinct pattern within the universe that is unique and essential to the tapestry of the whole. As MacIntyre (1984) asserted, the individual is understood within the context of a setting over time, and the narrative of any one life is part of an interlocking set of narratives (p. 218). There is support in the nursing literature for conceptualizing individuals in this way.

Barbara Sarter (1987) suggested that evolutionary idealism is an appropriate ontological basis for the development of nursing knowledge. Within this idealist worldview, human beings are seen as connected with the universe, all being of one fundamental nature, that of consciousness. The purpose of evolution is thought to be the unfolding of consciousness, the "refinement and development of cognition, volition, and emotion" (p. 5). Through the nurse, the individual client is said to find personal meaning in the experiences of health and illness. Moreover, Sarter held that the client is the final authority on what a life of quality means to him or her personally. Thus the individual is a source of truth, one aspect of the whole or unity of life.

Similarly, Margaret Newman's (1986) conceptualization of health as expanding consciousness is based on an ontology of consciousness unfolding and becoming manifest within the dynamic intercourse between the individual and the environment. In the introduction to the first edition of her book *Health as Expanding Consciousness,* Newman (1986) described her work as a synthesis of learning and experience. She acknowledged the importance of intuition in her life and stated, "There comes a time when one seeks knowledge that is more than the observable facts" (p. 5). She then referred to the work of David Bohm, a theoretical physicist whose theory of the invisible pattern or implicate order of the universe attested to her own experience that all of the universe is interconnected. According to this theory, whereas the implicate order is invisible, the explicate order is visible, consisting of the visible manifestations of energy transfer and boundaries imposed by our creation of time and space. Newman (1986) posited that each individual has a life pattern and that when this pattern is recognized and accepted, illness, suffering, and fear lose their power. Her theory is about the meaning of life and health.

The Individual as Part
of the Unity of Life

For the purposes of discussion, I offer a model of the individual as an open, conscious, and intelligent being whose "picture" can be taken at an intersection of time and space but who is really constantly changing. The individual, as depicted in Figure 4.1, has boundaries that define the physical self and psychological self as unique and distinct from that of other individuals.

The environment in which the individual exists flows into, and out of, the physical manifestation of consciousness that is the individual. As depicted in Figure 4.2, the individual is constantly exchanging energy with the universe. For example, as we breathe in air, we take in bits of the universe, and as we exhale, we return bits of ourselves

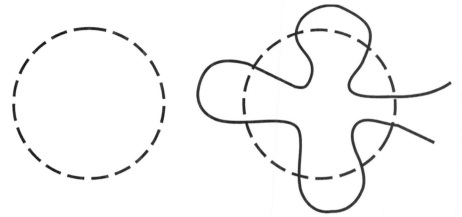

Figure 4.1. Individual   Figure 4.2. Individual-Environment

to the universe. The individual and the universe are thus one, a unity of life, a manifestation of energy.

Time and space are not real entities but inventions of human consciousness (see Figure 4.3). Deepak Chopra (1990) pointed out that more than 99% of our bodies is made up of empty spaces, which are not spaces of nothingness but spaces of pure conscious energy or

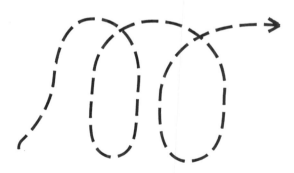

Figure 4.3. Time-Space

intelligence and potentiality. For Chopra, the same life energy that flows through the ocean throbs through our veins as well. In his view of the unity of life, in which all of the universe is thought to be connected through the empty spaces of intelligence and information, healing is emphasized.

A legendary tale from the Ayurvedic tradition of medicine as told by Kartha (1993) illustrates this unity of life. A student named Jeevaka was taking his final practical examination. The mentoring physician, Aatreya, directed the examinees to spend 1 week going into the heavily wooded hills around the medical school and to return with all the plants, animals, and minerals they could find that did not have any medicinal value. Aatreya's students quickly took to the hills with various tools for digging, scraping, sucking, and so forth. At the end of the week, students and teacher gathered in the school with an enormous variety of seeds, flowers, animal secretions, minerals, and other objects that the students believed had no medicinal qualities. Jeevaka, however, was the only student to return completely empty-handed. Aatreya, the teacher, asked, "Jeevaka, why have you brought nothing back from the hills? Have you decided not to take the exam?" Jeevaka replied,

> Revered Aatreya, I did the exercise as you instructed. I have searched for as long as I have studied with you and I found, as I have found before, that everything is filled with medicinal power: the animals, the plants, the songs of the birds, the shadows of the clouds, the sunlight and the wind. The omnipresence of healing is what I discovered today, as I have done before. Please evaluate my work on the basis of this answer. (p. 83)

Needless to say, Jeevaka had mastered the discipline and passed this test of medicine.

The Individual and the
Unity of Life in Nursing Inquiry

Like Jeevaka, we live in a healing universe that affirms the unity of life. In nursing, we often focus on the individual for the purpose of healing one who is not in harmony with the universe. We locate the

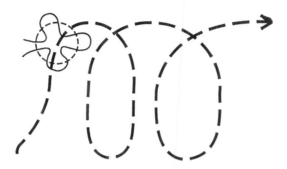

Figure 4.4. Snapshot of Individual-Environment at an Intersection in Time-Space

individual at a particular intersection in time and space, as shown in Figure 4.4, and engage in nursing inquiry to establish truths about the individual—those individuals who are our clients as well as those who are our colleagues. At times we expand our focus to include other individuals, those human beings closest to the client, such as their family members and friends, and those who make up the health care team with whom we work together for the client's well-being. But this has not always been the case.

Chopra (1990) contrasted an old paradigm of science in which humans are viewed as machines that learn to think with a new one in which humans are thought of as manifestations of intelligence. This analogy of humans as machines is applicable to the evolution of nursing science. In much of our formal research during the past four decades, we have conceptualized the individual as a machine, as adapting to an external environment. Only recently have we come to acknowledge what our practicing mentors knew long ago: The individual is interacting continuously with an ever-changing healing environment characterized by thought and intelligence. Our methods of inquiry have yielded facts about humans as machines while our practitioners have come to know and understand nursing's truths about human beings through meaningful healing experiences. An experience that I had during my first summer as a nursing assistant bears witness to this point. Further, it reveals the seeds of truth about nursing that were later to influence my philosophy, practice, and pursuit of knowledge in nursing.

A PERSONAL EXPERIENCE

Slightly more than 30 years ago, during the summer before I began my formal nursing education, I worked as a nursing assistant on the 3 to 11 p.m. shift at a nearby county hospital. Though I had grown up in a small farming community in southeastern Iowa where everyone knew everyone else and "their people," I knew very few people in the county seat where the hospital was located because it was situated more than 10 miles from my farm home. Thus, upon applying for the nursing assistant position, I was relieved to discover that the wife of our rural route postman, whom I will call Eve, was the charge nurse of the unit where I was to spend much of the next two summers.

During my introduction to the practice of nursing, I came face to face with many of the harsh realities that are typically associated with being a nurse: emptying filthy, smelly bedpans; soaking stained linens; scrubbing contaminated instruments; and finding an elderly gentleman dead in his wheelchair after dinner. Whenever my mother would run into Eve at the grocery store, Eve would apologize for not protecting me from these realities. However, my mother would smile and tell her not to worry, that I had been around plenty of messes in my young life and that I did not seem to be any the worse for the wear.

In addition to having my eyes opened to some of the harsh realities about nursing that summer and, admittedly, having some second thoughts about whether this was the route I wanted to take in terms of my life's work, I also had my consciousness opened to truths about individuals in nursing, nurses and clients (or patients, as we referred to them in the early 1960s) alike. In this regard, the most meaningful aspect of my summer experiences was the opportunity I had to witness, in the interactions between Eve (who soon became my mentor and idol) and a patient (whom I will call Mrs. Jensen), truths in nursing about the individual and the unity of life.

Mrs. Jensen was dying from cervical cancer so advanced that it had spread to her vulva and was slowly eating away at the inner aspects of her thighs. The sight of her wounds was horrible and indelibly printed on my young mind. The stench of her decaying body was nauseating despite the many cans of bathroom spray we used to mask the odor. Moving her even the slightest bit caused her to cry out in pain as her bones crackled from the metastasis of the disease. I watched everything that Eve did for Mrs. Jensen, and I listened to every instruction she gave me about why she was doing this or that as she irrigated Mrs. Jensen's wounds and applied the complex layers of dressings. Each time we entered Mrs. Jensen's room, I would test myself to determine whether I could remember exactly what steps Eve took in giving the prescribed treatments. After the first 2 to 3 weeks, I gave up this exercise because she never did exactly the same thing twice! In time, I stopped worrying about this and felt myself getting caught up in the rhythm Eve established as she entered Mrs. Jensen's room. Stopping to ask Mrs. Jensen's son about his infant daughter, or her son-in-law about the progress of the corn they had planted that spring, Eve never appeared to be in a hurry to complete her tasks or to check off all her duties on a predetermined list of doctor's orders.

What was different about Eve's care of Mrs. Jensen was the vital flow of energy that I felt when I accompanied her on her nightly missions. Mrs. Jensen was not that "poor cancer patient in Room 201"; she was a precious individual who cared deeply about her family, her church, and her community. Although I never heard her utter a word in the 2 months she was hospitalized that summer, I knew that Mrs. Jensen cared about her family and friends because that care came back to her in countless ways. I also felt the comfort that Eve provided to Mrs. Jensen and her family. Despite her own sense that there was little she could do for Mrs. Jensen and that perhaps she really should try to shield me from the atrocity of illness, Eve continued to nurse and to model truths about nursing to me through every fiber of her being.

Somehow, when I was in Mrs. Jensen's room with Eve, the boundaries that separated her from Mrs. Jensen, and Mrs. Jensen from me, and me from Eve, became very fuzzy. There was a unity of life in those moments that transcended the frightening sight of flesh decaying and the agonizing sounds of bones disintegrating. I could feel the connections among us as we worked, preparing Mrs. Jensen to manifest a different type of consciousness from the one she had known and expressed through her first 50-some years of living in the world. When Mrs. Jensen died, we all felt some relief as well as sadness. As a young nursing assistant, I felt that I had been touched by the very essence of eternity, although I could not articulate that at the time.

For two summers, I looked forward to my evenings in the company of Eve. I never saw her write a nursing care plan, nor did she state a nursing diagnosis. Her gentle and generous demeanor, however, seemed to bring a certain brightness and peacefulness to the environment wherever she went. What she taught me about the individual and the interconnectedness of nurse and client was never in any of the textbooks I read over the next decade of my undergraduate and graduate education in nursing. But her influence had been powerful and penetrated my defenses. Without being aware of it at the time, I had internalized a way of knowing that would be reflected in my life's work in the nursing profession.

A few years later, when I was a student in a baccalaureate nursing program, the things I had learned working with Eve became apparent in my work. For example, during my clinical evaluation at the end of the first semester, I was a bit taken aback when my instructor, with a stack of my nursing care plans on her desk, asked how I had come to write the things I had in my nursing care plans that were not reflective of content covered in class and in our texts. Hence she questioned whether I might be "intuitive." As a naive nursing student, I was not sure whether I was being criticized or mocked, and because I did not know the meaning of the word *intuitive*, I simply shrugged and replied that I did not know. In retrospect, I now recognize that I was probably no more intuitive than any other intelligent young woman in my class; rather, I had incorporated what I had learned from watching Eve and synthesized it with what I was currently learning in nursing school.

Years later, my early experiences in nursing became the springboard for my research into the phenomenon of intuition and its use in clinical nursing practice (Rew, 1986, 1990; Rew & Barrow, 1987). For me, intuition represents the unity of life expressed in consciousness.

What I came to know to be truths in nursing were the result of a creative synthesis of scientific facts and personal experience. It is knowing the whole of a phenomenon without reducing it into mutually exclusive parts. It is understanding the unity of living and healing through time without breaking the acts of caring into discrete, linear steps. Truth, known as a whole, goes beyond the limitations of mechanistic, linear thought, bringing together the wisdom from the past with possibilities for the future. Chopra (1990) noted that our "gut feelings" may be even more valid and reliable than our reasoned thought. Physiologically, the stomach makes the same potent chemicals, neuropeptides, as the brain. These neuropeptides communicate messages between cells; they are intelligent messengers. The difference between thinking in the brain and thinking in the stomach, according to Chopra, is that the stomach is more primitive. Because of this primitiveness, it has not learned to doubt itself as the brain has.

Summary and Conclusions

Mercury symbolizes, for me, the unity of life that I believe is a truth in nursing. The individual drops, in constant interaction with each other, at one moment appear separate and autonomous. In the next, they collide and collude, forming communities that appear to act as a whole, then separate, once again, into dozens of singular bodies scampering across a seemingly thoughtless and impenetrable surface.

Working with Eve was, for me, a quintessential example of the unity of life expressed in nursing. These were moments when thoughts, feelings, and actions all blended together as energy flowed between me and Eve, novice and expert nurse, and our client, Mrs. Jensen, creating evolutionary changes in each of us as individuals.

Let me try to convey, in poetic form, what I have attempted to convey in prose.

> From mercury spilled by a child
> Through a glimpse of eternity as a novice nurse
> To formal inquiry into the truth of intuition;
> Markers of evolution within a single nurse,
> Thought and reflection taking form,
> Ideas turned into words;
> What is truth in these ideas, thoughts, and words?
> Whence have they come?
> And where are they going?

References

Chopra, D. (1990). *Magical mind, magical body*. Niles, IL: Nightingale-Conant.

Henderson, V. (1966). *The nature of nursing*. New York: Macmillan.

Kartha, D. K. M. (1993). Jeevaka's test/Buddhist. *Parabola: The Magazine of Myth and Tradition, 18*, 82-83.

MacIntyre, A. (1984). *After virtue*. Notre Dame, IN: University of Notre Dame Press.

Meleis, A. I. (1991). *Theoretical nursing: Development and progress* (2nd ed.). Philadelphia: J. B. Lippincott.

Newman, M. A. (1986). *Health as expanding consciousness*. St. Louis: C. V. Mosby.

Nightingale, F. (1946). *Notes on nursing: What it is, and what it is not*. Philadelphia: J. B. Lippincott. (Original work published 1859)

Rew, L. (1986). Intuition: Concept analysis of a group phenomenon. *Advances in Nursing Science, 8*(2), 21-28.

Rew, L. (1990). Intuition in critical care nursing practice. *Dimensions of Critical Care Nursing, 9*(1), 30-37.

Rew, L., & Barrow, E. M. (1987). Intuition: A neglected hallmark of nursing knowledge. *Advances in Nursing Science, 10*(1), 49-62.

Sarter, B. (1987). Evolutionary idealism: A philosophical foundation for holistic nursing theory. *Advances in Nursing Science, 9*(2), 1-9.

CHAPTER 5

Community, Culture, and Truth in Nursing Inquiry

SHIRLEY CLOUTIER LAFFREY

Let me begin my discussion of community, culture, and truth in nursing inquiry with the story of the blindfolded children who were placed in a room with an elephant. When asked to explore and describe it, each child experienced a different aspect of the elephant and described that aspect as if it constituted the elephant in toto. Similarly, each of us has a different vantage point from which we view the "elephant" called nursing inquiry. Given this, it is vital to keep reminding ourselves that our individual views of the phenomenon of nursing inquiry are the perspectives each of us has of parts rather than the whole of it at a given moment. Add to this the notion that both perspectives and phenomenon are constantly interacting and evolving over time, and we begin to see the complexity of describing nursing inquiry. In my view, it is the ability to see the parts while not losing sight of the meaning of the whole, or of the interconnectedness of the parts within the evolving whole, that characterizes nursing.

The focus of nursing inquiry is the human being in interaction with the environment. The quest for a deeper understanding of the "human being-environment interaction" has been ongoing throughout the history of nursing. Nightingale (1859/1969) taught us the importance of considering the environment in the care of patients. She did not view nurses as healers; rather, she believed that healing was a natural process inherent in the individual's relationship with his or her environment. In her book *Notes on Nursing,* Nightingale spoke of the laws of health and deplored the lack of attention given to the "laws which God has assigned to the relations of our bodies with the world in which He has put them" (p. 11). Nursing was thus charged, by Nightingale, to attend to factors in the environment (e.g., water, air, and noise) and to remove obstacles to providing an environment harmonious with the natural healing process. These thoughts reflect Nightingale's concern with the influence of the immediate environment on the individual patient.

In this chapter, the individual-environment interaction is examined and the concepts of *community* and *culture* are addressed as indicators of environment and of the dynamic nature of truth in nursing inquiry. The question remains, however, whether the environment is a force that must be taken into consideration because of its influence on the client or whether the environment is a focus of inquiry for nursing in its own right. In discussing the environment, I begin with the premise that all of life is interconnected and continuous.

Interconnectedness and Continuity

The interconnectedness and continuity of life are described by Rogers (1970), who conceptualizes human beings and the environment as contiguous energy fields continuously interacting with one another and manifested by "concomitant and constant alterations in the patterning of both" (p. 64). Within the Rogerian perspective, no boundary is thought to exist between human beings and their environments in that "people and their environments are perceived as irreducible energy fields integral with one another and continuously creative in their evolution" (Rogers, 1986, p. 184). Hence viewing the patient or client separately from his or her environment is considered to be particularistic.

MacIntyre (1984) stated that

> in our modern world, human life is partitioned into segments, each with its own norms and modes of behaviour. Thus we separate private life from public life, leisure from work, and individual from community. In doing so, the focus becomes the distinctiveness of each concept rather than the pattern of unity that is formed by each pair of concepts. (p. 204)

MacIntyre went on to argue, "Particular actions derive their character as parts of larger wholes" (p. 205). Although this point of view is gaining prominence, nursing practice and research continue to be approached analytically, with life, health, and illness treated in a particularistic manner as if they were a series of discrete events.

Polanyi (1962) noted that one cannot attend to two levels of awareness at the same time and used as an example of this point the playing of a piece of music on the piano. He argued that when the pianist shifts his awareness to the particulars of his fingers touching the keyboard, his awareness of the pattern of the music is destroyed. Thus he asserted that "all particulars become meaningless if we lose sight of the pattern which they jointly constitute" (p. 57).

Similarly, when we view the individual as an entity separate from the environment, we lose sight of the patterning that makes the individual and his or her behavior intelligible. For example, if I walked up to you and said, "Mary started an exercise program this morning," what I said would probably not make sense to you. However, if you found out that I had mistaken you for the individual who had expressed concern the previous day about Mary's sedentariness and lack of exercise, then, in that context, my comment would make sense to you. Thus it is the context that gives meaning to particular words and actions and renders the unity of life visible. As Hanchett (1979) stated, if we fix our eyes only on the foreground, we do not see the background. The foreground is the individual, and the background is the spatial context of contemporaneous events within which the individual, inclusive of his or her behavior, is situated.

Events have a historical continuity as well as a connection with contemporaneous events. MacIntyre (1984) noted that "the setting [or context] has a history within which the histories of individual agents not only are, but have to be situated, just because without the setting and its changes through time, the history of the individual agent and his changes through time will be unintelligible" (p. 206). We make particular events intelligible by viewing them within the context of other, similar, previously encountered events. For example, the first time fire was observed, fire itself was probably meaningless as well as frightening. Likewise, the idea that beings from other planets exist within our midst is somewhat unintelligible to many people. However, as our history continues to unfold and as frightening and unusual events such as these continue to occur over time, meaning will be ascribed to them. Events, situations, and individuals can therefore be understood only within a spatial context of contemporaneous events that renders them intelligible and within a historical context that includes their continuity with prior events and their probable continuity with future events.

Interconnectedness, Continuity, and the Community

How, one might ask, do the concepts of interconnectedness and continuity relate to that of community? Although Nightingale is best known for her concern related to the care of the individual patient, she also functioned at the broader community level (Reed & Zurakowski, 1989), gathering statistics and advocating for community action to improve sanitation and to reduce mortality and morbidity. Though this aspect of her work is not as well publicized, Nightingale's concern with community action is evident in her claim that "one could better predict health problems if one inspected houses, conditions, and ways of life, rather than the physical body" (Nightingale, cited in Reed & Zurakowski, 1989, p. 38). In a similar vein, Milic (1976) noted that an individual's health status is a function of the availability of health-sustaining resources, that health-seeking patterns are related to perceptions of limited resources, that community-wide decisions determine the range of resources available, and that individual health-related decisions are influenced by efforts to maximize valued resources in both the personal and the societal domains. Thus she proposed that individuals must be considered within the context of the community and larger society.

Blum (1981) defined *community* as consisting of human beings living within a hierarchy of natural systems and *health* as a function of harmony in the interrelationships between levels of systems. Hanchett (1979), who also used a systems approach, noted that people in relationship to one another and in relationship to place, resources, and services are the focus of nursing research and nursing practice at the community level. She defined *community* as more than and different from the sum of its people or their interrelations (Hanchett, 1979, 1986). She posed the following questions concerning the community: "Do you feel energized or devitalized by being there? What is the level of fear, hope, spontaneity, joy, or sadness there? Is it a young, growing, vibrant community or is it mature and calm? Is it aging, and if so, is it aging well or is it decaying?" (Hanchett, 1979, p. 26). The health of the community is thus viewed as a function of the energy, individuality, and relationships of the community as a whole and of the individuals and groups within the community.

The need to consider the concept of community from a broad perspective is evident in Butterfield's (1990) description of a group of physicians who were so busy treating sick children that they never took the time to determine what conditions within the community might be contributing to their illness. This "band-aid" approach, which she calls "downstream thinking," is all too common in our health care system. In contrast to this, an example of the effectiveness of community-focused care is to be found in the east side of the city in which I currently reside. The neighborhood in that section of the city is characterized by high rates of unemployment, poverty, violence, and sickness among the residents, many of whom have inadequate (or no) health insurance or health care. As well, several oil companies have gasoline and oil storage tanks underground, directly beneath or in close proximity to the residents' homes. These storage tanks have been there for many years, and until a year ago no one questioned the effect of the tanks on the health of this community. Then someone asked whether the high level of illness in the community might be related to the tanks. The people in the community began to demand that the air and soil be tested for toxic chemicals and that action be taken to reduce potential risks to the community. As a result of this community action, the oil companies have agreed to remove the tanks. This example serves to illustrate that acting at the community level to find and treat a problem at its source can produce greater, more far-reaching health benefits than simply treating manifestations of an illness in individuals that may be the result of a larger problem.

Individuals make choices about their health practices, but the degree to which they can exercise their freedom to make personal health choices is affected by other individuals, their families, available options, and the norms and values of the community. No longer can we delude ourselves into thinking that lasting behavior change will take place by intervening at the individual level without also intervening at the immediate and surrounding community level. Chopoorian (1986) stated that our lack of consciousness related to community may account for nursing's peripheral role in the larger arena of health care.

From early nursing times to the present day we, as nurses, have become increasingly aware that we must consider community as one indicator of environment if the care that we provide is to be optimally effective in its impact on health. Brandon (1983) noted that in the old paradigm of health care within the community, the highest level of development is thought to be development of the self, with individual health viewed as a concern with the self. However, Wilbur (1980) contrasted this approach with a new paradigm that emphasizes unity with a greater whole. In this new paradigm, previously dichotomized states, such as love and hate, rationality and irrationality, and individual and community, give way to a unity and a synthesis that moves beyond and is greater than each of the dichotomized parts. Edwards and Dees (1990) supported this new paradigm approach, stating that the contribution of nursing to the community's health lies in nursing's ability to integrate health and disease, individual and group, and public health and nursing.

Today, as more and more nursing care is being provided outside the acute care arena, it is more important than ever that we, as nurses, develop a clear understanding of human-environment interactions as

a basis for undertaking health promotion, illness and disability prevention, and illness-related care in the community. However, in addition to community, nurses must also consider culture as an important
indicator of environment.

Interconnectedness, Continuity, and Culture

Culture has become of increasing concern to nursing, primarily
due to the increase in cultural diversity, not just within our large
cities but within our small towns and rural areas as well. As Meleis
(1992) identified, "There is an increasing tendency among minorities,
refugees and immigrants to maintain home country or ancestral
cultural heritage" (p. 152). The resulting variety in languages
spoken, lifestyles, and expression of values and needs has forced
nursing to acknowledge the cultural diversity that exists within our
communities.

But what is culture? As was noted previously, culture and community are being considered as indicators of environment in this chapter.
Leininger (1985) used the terms *culture* and *environment* synony-
mously and defined culture as the "learned, shared, and transmitted
values, beliefs, norms, and lifeway practices of a particular group that
guides thinking, decisions, and actions in patterned ways" (p. 209).
She noted that studying an individual without reference to the environmental or cultural context limits a full and accurate understanding
of that human being. Because an individual cannot be considered
separately from the environment and because culture is a characteristic
of the individual, culture is a fundamental manifestation of the human-environment interaction.

Culture can also be viewed as a dynamic pattern of people's relationships to each other and to the place, resources, and services within
a given community (Hanchett, 1979, 1986). The unique pattern of
these relationships is the culture of the community and is a reflection
of the expanding consciousness of the community and its people.

Conclusion

Marchione (1986, p. 110) cited Bohm's (1983, p. 35) idea that "individuals and communities must be viewed as interconnected and relational, as undivided and whole" and that the word *individual* means "undivided." It is thus not possible to have true individuality except when individuality is grounded in the whole. Bohm's perspective is not unlike the unitary-transformative perspective proposed by Newman, Sime, and Corcoran-Perry (1991), in which each individual is thought to be a self-organizing field embedded in a larger, self-organizing field. There is an interpenetration of fields within fields, with the whole moving in the direction of greater complexity.

As MacIntyre (1984) noted, when attention is paid to the dynamic interplay of the individual client and the community, the health situation becomes intelligible. The individual is situated within a spatial context of contemporaneous events, experiences, beliefs, and perceptions and is situated at the same time within a historical context of all past and potential future life events, experiences, beliefs, and perceptions. The point and time at which the spatial and historical contexts intersect constitute the explicit health situation that is presented to us, as nurses, by the individual.

If we attend only to what is explicit, we may restrict our care to individualistic, short-term, "band-aid" solutions. Alternatively, broadening our perspective to include the larger, dynamic patterning of the interrelations of the individual, culture, and community can lead to long-term solutions for the individual as well as for the environment with which the individual is coextensive. This broader approach to nursing acknowledges the unity and interconnectedness of life, which is reflected in what characterizes nursing: the ability to view the individual while not losing sight of the unity of the whole or of the interconnectedness of the parts within the evolving whole.

References

Blum, H. L. (1981). *Planning for health* (2nd ed.). New York: Human Sciences Press.

Bohm, D. (1983). Of matter and meaning: The superimplicate order. A conversation between David Bohm and Renee Weber. *Re-Vision, 6*(1), 34-44.

Brandon, N. (1983). *Honoring the self: Personal integrity and the heroic potentials.* Los Angeles: Tarcher.

Butterfield, P. G. (1990). Thinking upstream: Nurturing a conceptual understanding of the societal context of health behaviour. *Advances in Nursing Science, 12*(2), 1-8.

Chopoorian, T. J. (1986). Reconceptualizing the environment. In P. Moccia (Ed.), *New approaches to theory development* (pp. 39-54). New York: National League for Nursing.

Edwards, L. H., & Dees, R. L. (1990). Environmental health: The effects of life-style on the world around us. In S. J. Wold (Ed.), *Community health nursing: Issues and topics* (pp. 231-266). Norwalk, CT: Appleton & Lange.

Hanchett, E. S. (1979). *Community health assessment.* New York: John Wiley.

Hanchett, E. S. (1986). *Nursing frameworks and community as client.* Norwalk, CT: Appleton & Lange.

Leininger, M. (1985). Transcultural care diversity and universality: A theory of nursing. *Nursing and Health Care, 6*(4), 209-212.

MacIntyre, A. (1984). *After virtue* (2nd ed.). Notre Dame, IN: University of Notre Dame Press.

Marchione, J. M. (1986). Application of the new paradigm of health to individuals, families, and communities. In M. A. Newman (Ed.), *Health as expanding consciousness* (pp. 107-134). St. Louis: C. V. Mosby.

Meleis, A. I. (1992). Cultural diversity research. *Communicating Nursing Research, 25,* 151-173.

Milio, N. (1976). A framework for prevention: Changing health-damaging to health-generating patterns. *American Journal of Public Health, 66,* 435-439.

Newman, M. A., Sime, M., & Corcoran-Perry, S. A. (1991). The focus of the discipline of nursing. *Advances in Nursing Science, 14*(1), 1-6.

Nightingale, F. (1969). *Notes on nursing: What it is and what it is not.* New York: Dover. (Original work published 1859)

Polanyi, M. (1962). *Personal knowledge: Towards a post-critical philosophy.* Chicago: University of Chicago Press.

Reed, P. G., & Zurakowski, T. L. (1989). Nightingale revisited: A visionary model for nursing. In J. J. Fitzpatrick & A. L. Whall (Eds.), *Conceptual models of nursing: Analysis and application* (pp. 33-47). Norwalk, CT: Appleton & Lange.

Rogers, M. E. (1970). *An introduction to the theoretical basis of nursing.* Philadelphia: F. A. Davis.

Rogers, M. E. (1986). Science of unitary human beings. In V. Malinski (Ed.), *Explorations of Martha Rogers' science of unitary human beings* (pp. 3-7). Norwalk, CT: Appleton-Century-Crofts.

Wilbur, K. (1980). The pre/trans fallacy. *Re-Vision, 3*(2), 51-72.

CHAPTER 6

Traditions, Rationality, and Truth in Nursing Inquiry

JOY HINSON PENTICUFF

In pursuing truth in nursing, we must consider several questions. How ought we to decide which accounts of truth in nursing deserve our allegiance? How should we choose among competing accounts of what it means to do good in nursing? And how do our modes of inquiry and our traditions combine to produce views of the world that are consistent with our experiences in nursing? In exploring answers to these questions and in describing nursing traditions, I draw from the work of Alasdair MacIntyre (1984, 1988) and use his notion of traditions as the shared attitudes, beliefs, presuppositions, and modes of inquiry characteristic of a discipline. I also use Charles Schunior's (1989) poetic descriptions of the donning of tragic and comic masks to illustrate how nursing's traditions, rationality, and inquiry have changed in the past quarter century.

Rational Inquiry and
Justification Within Traditions

MacIntyre (1988) held that the concepts of rationality and justification cannot be understood outside the contextual framework of the individual in his or her roles within a social and cultural tradition. He asserted that "there is no standing ground, no place for inquiry, no way to engage in the practices of advancing, evaluating, accepting, and rejecting reasoned argument apart from that which is provided by some particular tradition or other" (p. 350). The postmodern conception of ideal rationality, which consists of principles attained by a socially disembodied being, illegitimately ignores that principles of rationality, whether theoretical or practical, are historically and socially context bound (p. 4).

MacIntyre (1988) asserted that the postmodernist rationality, which requires that we "abstract ourselves from all those particulars of social relationship in terms of which we have been accustomed to understand our responsibilities and our interests," will result in "conceptions of universality and impersonality which . . . are far too thin and meagre to supply what is needed" (p. 334). Hence any rationality that requires a neutral, impartial, and universal point of view cannot adequately depict the reality of persons within relationships and contexts. This view affirms, for nursing, the necessity of seeing persons in their situations and recognizing the emergent qualities of those situations.

RATIONAL INQUIRY WITHIN TRADITIONS

For MacIntyre (1988), the history of a particular form of rational inquiry cannot be isolated from the collective life narratives of the adherents to the convictions within a tradition. "Theories of rationality confront us as aspects of traditions, allegiance to which requires the living out of human life, with its specific modes of social relationship, canons of interpretation and evaluation in respect of the behaviour of others, each with its own evaluative practices" (p. 391).

MacIntyre (1988) characterized the traditions of rational inquiry as sets of shared attitudes, beliefs, and presuppositions that are developed in a different way within each particular tradition, affording different and incompatible answers to questions. From the plurality of traditions, multiple rationalities emerge—persons within one tradition reason differently from those within another tradition because of variations in linguistics, historical context, experience, and so forth. This is evident in the various understandings about the patient held by the nurse, physician, psychologist, social worker, and chaplain, which are reflective of the different reasoning processes and modes of inquiry characteristic of each discipline. However, MacIntyre also held that the diversity of traditions of rational inquiry and justification does not preclude rational resolution of differences between rival and incompatible traditions. "The problem of diversity is not abolished, but is transformed in a way that renders it amenable of solution" (p. 10). Convictions can be justified and traditions maintained or rejected by means of internal and external analyses of convictions within traditions.

JUSTIFICATION OF
CONVICTIONS WITHIN TRADITIONS

A major feature of MacIntyre's (1988) analysis of convictions is the use of forms of rational inquiry through which "correspondence between what the mind judges and believes and reality as perceived, classified, and understood" (p. 356) is affirmed. Thus, through practical reasoning within a particular tradition, the ideas formulated and accepted as true by adherents of that tradition are vindicated as rationally superior to competing ideas because they can be shown, through dialectical questioning, to be adequate and accurate conceptions of the reality of life within that tradition. Throughout the history of the tradition, the adequacy and accuracy of the tradition's intellectual resources in conceptualizing human experience justify allegiance to the tradition.

It is important to understand the way in which MacIntyre (1988) characterized the activities of the intellect in the process of rational justification within traditions. It is his contention that the intellect is not to be conceived of as a Cartesian mind or a materialist brain. Rather, it ought to be conceptualized as that through which individuals relate to each other and to natural and social objects as these are presented to them (p. 355). Thus his conception of rationality and truth in traditions is at odds with both the Cartesian and the Hegelian accounts of rationality in that rational justification is based, not on principles that are acceptable to all rational persons, but rather on the superiority of formulations of ideas as compared with previous formulations of them held by adherents of a particular tradition (Post, 1989, p. 49).

For MacIntyre (1988), ideas used to characterize human experience within traditions, and the convictions that these ideas support, are subject to verification (in the case of ideas) and justification (in the case of convictions) through practical reasoning. Because the lives of persons within traditions are not static, changing realities require ongoing analysis of whether the ideas and convictions to which people within a tradition adhere are worthy of the allegiance given. Rational inquiry provides the justification for giving allegiance to, or rejecting, ideas and convictions and by implication evaluates the rational superiority or inferiority of the tradition itself in comparison with other traditions. In addition, within each tradition "the standards of rational justification themselves emerge from and are part of a history in which they are vindicated by the way in which they transcend the limitations of and provide remedies for the defects of their predecessors within the history of that same tradition" (p. 7).

MacIntyre (1988) described the rationality of a tradition in terms of the progress it makes through three stages of maturation. First is the stage of settled conviction, in which the beliefs, institutions, and practices of some particular community are taken as givens. Authority is conferred upon certain texts and voices, and these are deferred to without systematic questioning. However, because all communities are in a state of change and because human lives, and therefore traditions, are open systems capable of perceiving and responding to the ideas and convictions of other worldviews, the authority of some beliefs begins to be doubted. In this second stage, events may challenge existing characterizations of reality, bringing into question accepted ideas and convictions. When this happens, authoritative texts or utterances are seen as susceptible to alternative and incompatible interpretations, enjoining incompatible courses of action. Incoherences in the established system of beliefs may become evident, and confrontation by new situations, engendering new questions, may reveal a lack of resources for offering or for justifying answers to these new questions (MacIntyre, 1988, pp. 354-355).

It is not until persons within a tradition are able to recognize the correspondence of belief with reality that new ideas, convictions, and traditions can be seen to be superior to rival ideas, convictions, and traditions. This occurs in MacIntyre's (1988) third stage of development of a tradition. In this stage, those members of a community who have accepted the beliefs of the tradition in their new form become able to contrast their new beliefs with the old. There is a recognition of a "radical discrepancy" or lack of correspondence between the dominant beliefs of their own tradition and the reality disclosed by the newer, more successful explanations; thus the claim to truth of their former beliefs has been defeated. "It is this lack of correspondence, between what the mind then judged and believed and reality as now perceived, classified, and understood, which is ascribed when those earlier judgments and beliefs are called false" (p. 356). In this manner, the beliefs of a tradition can be rationally discredited by appeal to the tradition's very own standards of rationality. It is through the process of asserting the superiority of the new conception of reality that the relativist denial of the possibility of rational choice among rival traditions is defeated.

MacIntyre's (1988) characterization of the activities of the mind in determining falsity is instructive. The mind engages with objects in the natural and social world in terms of such activities as identification, reidentification, collecting, separating, classifying, and naming by touching, grasping, pointing, breaking down, building up, calling to, answering to, and so forth. As a result of its engagement with objects, the mind is informed by images that are or are not adequate (for the mind's purposes) representations of the particular objects or sorts of objects that are encountered and by concepts that are or are not adequate representations of the forms in terms of which the objects are grasped and classified. The mind is adequate to its objects insofar as the expectations that it frames on the basis of its activities are not liable to disappointment and insofar as the remembering in which it engages enables it to return to and recover what it had encountered previously, whether the objects themselves are still present or not.

Falsity is recognized when thought is not adequate in its dealings with the realities of the social and rational world (MacIntyre, 1988, pp. 355-357). With regard to truth, MacIntyre (1988) stated,

> To claim truth for one's present mind-set and the judgments which are its expression is to claim that this kind of inadequacy, this kind of discrepancy, will never appear in any possible future situation, no matter how searching the inquiry, no matter how much evidence is provided, no matter what developments in rational inquiry may occur. (p. 358)

> Thus there is a conception of a final truth, a relationship of the mind to its objects which would be wholly adequate in respect of the capacities of that mind. But there is no Absolute Knowledge as sought by the Hegelian system and no one at any stage can ever rule out the future possibility of their present beliefs and judgments being shown to be inadequate. (p. 361)

At each stage of development, tradition-constituted inquiry can be evaluated in terms of its adequacy in resolving conflicts. If hitherto adequate conceptualizations and methods of inquiry become sterile and practical principles come to be recognized as false, the tradition faces what MacIntyre (1988) termed an "epistemological crisis." This crisis can be successfully resolved through the innovative development of new concepts and theories that furnish a systematic and coherent solution to previously intractable problems; explain what rendered the tradition sterile or incoherent; and exhibit, in their solutions and explanations, some fundamental continuity between the new conceptual and theoretical structures and the previously held shared beliefs of the tradition (p. 362). Furthermore, if the tradition is to survive such an epistemological crisis, three other requirements must be met. First, because the concepts and theories that come into being are not derivable from earlier positions, conceptual innovation is necessary for the successful resolution of the crisis. Second, justification of the new concepts and theories must be based on their ability to achieve what could not have been achieved prior to that innovation. Finally, some core of shared belief, constitutive of allegiance to the tradition, must survive each crisis (MacIntyre, 1988).

It is apparent that some traditions have conceptual resources that are more adequate than those of others for constructing representations of the entirety of human experiencing. In terms of MacIntyre's (1988) account that successful resolution of epistemological crisis is dependent on the innovative capacities of persons within traditions, nursing is in a favorable position. This is because its traditions of inquiry are diverse, drawn from many sources within the social and natural sciences, enriched by creative synthesis, and focused through humanitarian lenses. Our traditions in nursing provide conceptual tools for evaluating the intelligibility of our practices and traditions.

Intelligibility in Nursing Traditions and Practices

MacIntyre (1984) defined a living tradition—as opposed to an archaic, ineffectual tradition—as "an historically extended, socially embodied argument about the goods which constitute that tradition" (p. 222). He noted that the history of a practice is embedded in, and made intelligible in terms of, the larger and longer history of the tradition through which the practice in its present form was conveyed to us. All nursing inquiry takes place within the context of nursing's traditional modes of thought. Nursing practices have histories, and, at any given moment, what nursing practice is depends on a mode of understanding that has been transmitted through many generations.

I believe that nursing's traditional modes of understanding have long embraced entering into experiences with a patient and focusing on the narrative of each patient's life so as to allow for an intelligible answer to the question "What is good for this patient?" However, our recent elevation of the scientific as the paramount mode of understanding has thrust us into an epistemological crisis. I will illustrate this by recalling the narrative presented, in Chapter 4 of this volume, by Rew of her experience as a novice nursing student learning from an expert nurse named Eve. The mode of understanding, or tradition, operant in this situation was that of our most recent past generation of expert nurses. The contrast between how the expert nurse reacted to a patient's pain 30 years ago and how the expert nurse would react today is indicative of an epistemological crisis that has occurred within the tradition of nursing. That difference reveals that a profound shift has taken place in how nurses view their role in terms of doing good for the patient, in this case Mrs. Jensen. To quote from Rew:

> Mrs. Jensen was dying from cervical cancer so advanced that it had spread to her vulva and was slowly eating away at the inner aspects of her thighs. The sight of her wounds was horrible and indelibly printed on my young mind. The stench of her decaying body was nauseating despite the many cans of bathroom spray we used to mask the odor. *Moving her even the slightest bit caused her to cry out in pain as her bones crackled from the metastasis of disease* [italics added]. . . What was different about Eve's care of Mrs. Jensen was the vital flow of energy that I felt when I accompanied her on her nightly missions. . . . I also felt the comfort that Eve provided to Mrs. Jensen and her family. . . . Eve continued to nurse and to model truths about nursing to me through every fiber of her being. . . . There was a unity of life in those moments that transcended the frightening sight of flesh decaying and the agonizing sounds of bones disintegrating. I could feel the connections among us as we worked, preparing Mrs. Jensen to manifest a different type of consciousness from the one she had known and expressed through her first 50-some years of living in the world.

In examining the above narrative, I am doing so not to deny the caring and healing inherent in Eve's interactions with Mrs. Jensen but to show that our understanding of what is good for a patient and the implications of that understanding have changed radically in the past quarter century. Today, in nursing, we see questioning of a care plan that does not include adequate pain management as essential to our role; 30 years ago, we did not. Eve, for all her compassion, did not see her role as one of advocating pain relief for a terminally ill patient. Such a shift in understanding with regard to patient good and the role of the nurse comes about as a result of an epistemological crisis within traditions. The crisis in question arose because of a lack of correspondence between what nurses saw themselves as able to do to accomplish patient good and what patient good truly demanded of nurses. In regard to relieving pain, Eve's compassion and nursing's traditional practices were in conflict; however, Eve did not recognize that she could do more. As MacIntyre (1984) eloquently put it,

> What the individual is able to do and say intelligibly . . . is deeply affected by the fact that we are never more (and sometimes less) than the co-authors of our own narratives. Only in fantasy do we live what story

we please. In life . . . we are always under certain constraints. We enter upon a stage which we did not design and find ourselves part of an action that was not of our making. Each of us being a main character in his own drama plays subordinate parts in the dramas of others, and each drama constrains the others. (p. 213)

MacIntyre concludes, shortly thereafter in the same book, that "the story of my life is always embedded in the story of those communities from which I derive my identity" (p. 221).

As individuals, we enter onto the stage of nursing. We are part of a social contract in which we play roles as helpers and coadventurers in dramas of the human condition. In each drama, there is both a shared reality and an isolated, exclusive reality: truth validated by its consistency across the experiences of the group and truth validated by its consistency across an individual life. The notion of "truth for the individual" can be understood in terms of some conception of the unity of a person's life (MacIntyre, 1988). In nursing, "truth for the individual" has to do with understanding the harmonies and discordancies of each patient's life. What is better or worse for the patient depends upon the character of the intelligible narrative that provides the patient's life with its unity.

I am constrained, as a nurse, by the actions of others and by the social setting presupposed in my own and others' actions.

At any point we do not know what will happen next, but this unpredictability coexists with a certain teleological character—certain conceptions of a possible future. In this future that we conceive of, certain possibilities beckon us forward and others repel us, some seem already foreclosed and others perhaps inevitable. There is no present which is not informed by some image of some future and . . . a variety of ends or goals towards which we are either moving or failing to move in the present. Unpredictability and teleology therefore coexist as parts of our lives; like characters in a fictional narrative, we do not know what will happen next, but nonetheless our lives have a certain form which projects itself towards our future. . . . If the narrative of our individual and social lives is to continue intelligibly—and either type of narrative may lapse into unintelligibility—it is always the case that there are constraints on how the story can continue and that within those constraints there are indefinitely many ways that it can continue. I can only answer the question "What am I to do?" if I can answer the prior question "Of what story or stories do I find myself a part?" (MacIntyre, 1984, pp. 215-216)

The work of Charles Schunior (1989) illustrates more clearly the differences in our modes of understanding patient good 30 years ago and our evolving modes of understanding patient good today. Schunior referred to Pearce's notions of the existence of multiple worlds, each exclusively "real" to each patient. He noted, "Our medically oriented therapeutic perspective is exclusively real to us but may compete or even conflict with our patients' world views" (p. 9).

Eve's perspective was to care for Mrs. Jensen, and she did so with every fiber of her being. But Eve's reality was a medical treatment orientation that excluded a full recognition of Mrs. Jensen's reality—the reality of agonizing pain and terminal illness. Indeed, because of her view of her role, Eve was less concerned with relieving pain than with masking odors. The provision of adequate pain relief was precluded because of the reality of nurse and physician, with its therapeutic orientation that agony was better than addiction and that life under any circumstances was better than death. Thus Eve's understanding within that archaic tradition of nursing was that the nurse must not depress the life force with high doses of narcotics and must not degrade the patient's character by engendering addiction. Rather, the nurse must compassionately turn the patient and change his or her dressings, all the while closing his or her ears, if possible, to the patient's moans and screams. The nurse must shut out his or her understanding of the pain that is "exclusively real" to the patient. Schunior (1989) lamented nursing's modern donning of the tragic mask and stated,

> The tragic hero is the character who is sure of his purpose and unswerving to the purpose no matter what the odds. The tragic hero has perceived a mandate to master experience. . . . The comic hero, on the other hand, seeks not to master experience but to "sink into its episodes." (pp. 10-11)

As nurses, we have taken on a worldview in which the chief mode of inquiry is thought to be scientific. We have learned to value understanding that allows for prediction and control of events and have adopted the model of scientific knowledge, predictability, and the if-then constant conjunction.

Fundamental to all of this is the dialogue between predicting, controlling, and intervening, on the one hand, and touching, apprehending, and feeling, on the other. In Schunior's (1989) words,

Curing . . . is a mechanical, functional restoration. But because fatality, loss, and change are the inescapable substrates of our existence, an exclusive emphasis on cure is necessarily frustrated and tragic. Healing also involves restoration, but in an existential rather than functional mode, a restoration to the centre of one's being. . . . Accepting patients as they are, where they are, without the tragic hero's concern with defining, controlling, and changing, permits the spirit to expand and express itself. (pp. 15-16)

In the case of Mrs. Jensen's "exclusive reality," which included suffering and terminal illness, we were sure of our roles as nurses: to change dressings and to fight off the Grim Reaper. Our therapeutic worldview precluded "sinking into the episodes" of her suffering and thus precluded relief of that suffering.

Conclusion

Rew's compelling example, in this volume, of nursing's traditions and worldview 30 years ago gives us a sense of how our discipline's perspective, self-definition, and emerging willingness to enter into the patient's reality are producing an increasingly truthful understanding of what is good for the patient and what our role may be as coadventurers toward that potential good. We are in the midst of epistemological change, a change that will be described in the next decade or so as nursing's affirmation of feeling, apprehending, and touching and of having put aside the tragic mask.

References

MacIntyre, A. (1984). *After virtue* (2nd ed.). Notre Dame, IN: University of Notre Dame Press.
MacIntyre, A. (1988). *Whose justice? Which reality?* Notre Dame, IN: University of Notre Dame Press.
Post, S. G. (1989). Tradition and practical reasoning: MacIntyre's dissent. *Medical Humanities Review, 3*(1), 48-50.
Schunior, C. (1989). Nursing and the comic mask. *Holistic Nursing Practice, 3*(3), 7-17.

CHAPTER 7

The Nature of Nursing: Natural or Conventional?

ANNE H. BISHOP

Is the nature of nursing natural or conventional? According to some, nursing's nature is natural; it has an essence that does not change and is to be discovered over time. In contrast, others hold that nursing is changing over time; its nature is to be developed and is conventional. In this chapter, I examine these distinctions and attempt to answer the question posed, from within the phenomenological tradition—the tradition within which I work. I begin by translating, as best as I can, the terms *natural* and *conventional* into phenomenological language.

Phenomenological Interpretation of Terms

In the phenomenological tradition, the notion of the nature of nursing as natural comes closest to Husserl's (1911/1965) notion of essential meaning, although Husserl would probably object violently to nursing's nature being labeled as *natural*. Husserl believed that by bracketing theories we can encounter things in and of themselves and lift out their essential meaning. It is claimed by some interpreters of Husserl's work that this approach was reflective of a new form of idealism in that it attempted to disclose an ahistorical essence. That aside, Husserl, late in his career, introduced the notion of *life world*, giving a historical dimension to the notion of meaning. Heidegger (1962) expanded Husserl's approach by contending that the human being is being-in-time; meaning, therefore, is to be disclosed by historical interpretation. John Scudder and I (Bishop & Scudder, 1990, 1991) have used both approaches and think that they work well together. Given this, I would eliminate the "or" in the question "Is the nature of nursing natural or conventional?" Further, I would take *natural* to mean "essential" and *conventional* to mean "being-in-time" or "historical."

If we were unable to "lift out" the essence of an activity, such as nursing, it would have no recognizable meaning. But if it were claimed that essence remains the same for all time, real historical development would be impossible. Yet if meanings were merely a matter of historical development, then, over time, practices might come to mean the opposite of what they originally meant. For example, suppose that nurses became technicians who merely took bodily measurements and entered them into a computer that then dictated what chemicals to give or what technological gadgets to attach to the patient. Would it not be intellectually more honest to say that medical technology had made nursing obsolete, rather than to continue to call such medical technologists nurses? Along this line of thought, consider the point made by Edmund Pellegrino, Director of the Kennedy Institute for Ethics at Georgetown University, that there are now many medical technicians who falsely call themselves physicians (personal communication, 1983). These physicians have become so involved with technological interventions that they have lost the sense of care for patients. As we all know, nursing has moved in a similar direction. However, despite this, let us see if we can "lift out" an essential meaning of nursing that is reflective of both contemporary nursing and Florence Nightingale's interpretation of nursing.

Essential Meaning of Nursing

Without considering the historical roots of nursing, it is not possible to determine whether there is an essence of nursing to be discovered over time or whether nursing has changed so much that it is a new entity, with a nature yet to be developed. Although there were references to nursing before the time of Florence Nightingale, nursing as the profession we know it to be had its beginnings with Nightingale. So let us begin with Nightingale.

In *Notes on Nursing,* Florence Nightingale (1859/1946) wrote, "If a patient is cold, if a patient is feverish, if a patient is faint, if he is sick after taking food, if he has a bed-sore, it is generally the fault not of the disease, but of the nursing. I use the word nursing for want of a better" (p. 6). She went on to say that nursing "ought to signify the proper use of fresh air, light, warmth, cleanliness, quiet, and the proper selection and administration of diet—all at the least expense of vital power to the patient" (p. 6). Thus, for Nightingale, it would seem that the essence of nursing was fostering healing and health through care.

Some nurses who work in the clean, air-conditioned environment of hospitals may not consciously think about the necessity of the elements, such as fresh air, mentioned by Nightingale. However, as community health nurses are well aware, they are no less important for health today than they were during the 1800s. Although nursing today entails more than the list of activities that Nightingale includes in her description of nursing, and although other definitions of nursing may be preferred to that of Nightingale, I believe that her definition is sufficiently well accepted to allow us to say that nursing can have an essential meaning over time.

Let us examine an example of contemporary nursing to see if Nightingale's definition of nursing as fostering healing and health through care makes sense. In so doing, we will be following phenomenological practice in conveying essential meaning through a well-chosen example (Ricoeur, 1977). The following story about JoAnn was related to me by Brenda, a registered nurse who works as the patient care coordinator at a private free clinic in Virginia.

JoAnn had been receiving her health care at one of the county health departments. She has a family history of insulin-dependent diabetes. I think her mother and father were both insulin dependent, but she had never been diagnosed as having diabetes. She came down here one night. I am not sure why she came here instead of continuing her care at the health department; maybe it was because the health department couldn't provide the medications she needed. She came down here and really didn't have any specific complaints. But since she was a first-time patient, we decided to do some baseline labs on her. So we did a chem screen.

The next morning when I came back to work, the lab at the hospital called and said, "I think you need to know that this lady has a blood sugar of over 900." I said, "As far as we know, she is not diabetic." I called the doctor who had seen her the night before. He said she needed to be in the emergency room so she could be admitted as an unassigned patient and started on insulin. So I called her. When nobody answered, I left a message on her answering machine asking her to call me right away. A few minutes later, she returned my phone call. I told her, "I don't want to frighten you, JoAnn, but you had a really, really high blood sugar, and the doctor who saw you last night would like you to go over to the emergency room because he thinks you need to be started on some medicine to bring that sugar under control." She got her husband to take her over there. A few days later, she came down to the clinic with her prescription in hand to get her insulin and her syringes. She had been admitted to the hospital, had been put on insulin, and had had diabetic teaching. She said, "Brenda, I just want to tell you that if you hadn't called when you did, I might not be here. I was feeling so bad that I was getting ready to go to bed and take a nap. By the time I got to the emergency room, my sugar was over 1,100. The doctors told me that if I had gone to sleep, I probably wouldn't have woken up. I would have gone into a coma. Your phone call came at just the right time."

Well, you can imagine what that did to my ego! I started thinking about what might have happened had I disregarded the lab's phone message, thinking, "I'll do it later," as everybody does—you get busy or distracted or whatever. She might very well have gone into a coma and never come out of it, or at least suffered terrible consequences. I enrolled her in our diabetic clinic last week. Her blood sugar had been running very good. When she was here last, it was 122. She knows all about diabetes because of her family history and having to give insulin to her mother and father and is doing all the right things for herself.

I will interpret Brenda's story in light of the three essentials of nursing that John Scudder and I disclosed in our books on nursing

(Bishop & Scudder, 1990, 1991). In so doing, I will attempt to show that Brenda's narrative of her nursing care, as well as Nightingale's (1859/1946) description of nursing, is consistent with these three essentials. The first is that nursing is a practice; the second, that nursing has a moral sense; and the third, that nursing is a practice of caring.

NURSING AS A PRACTICE

According to Alasdair MacIntyre's (1984) definition of a practice, nursing can be interpreted as a practice, a "coherent and complex form of socially established cooperative human activity" (p. 187). In a similar vein, the American Nurses' Association (1980) stated, in *Nursing: A Social Policy Statement,* that

> nursing, like other professions, is an essential part of the society out of which it grew and with which it has been evolving. Nursing can be said to be owned by society, in the sense that nursing's professional interest must be perceived as serving the interests of the larger whole of which it is a part. (p. 3)

But although a practice develops within a sociocultural context, it is the practitioners who develop the practice itself (MacIntyre, 1984).

MacIntyre (1984) stated that certain goods are accomplished through meeting the standards of excellence of a practice. Nightingale thought that the good was accomplished when nurses put the body in the best condition for healing. It is my opinion that Brenda probably also believes that. To put the body in the best condition for healing, she had to get JoAnn to the hospital to obtain the insulin she required and the teaching she needed to learn how to care for herself.

So how does Brenda's practice compare with that of a nurse who might have practiced in Nightingale's era? Today nurses have much more legitimate authority over their own practice. Brenda, as the only direct care health professional during the day in the clinic where she works, makes many decisions about her nursing practice as well as decisions about whether the patient requires care within the realm of medical practice. The skills and competencies that nurses such as Brenda exercise today often do not look like those of the 1950s, much less of the 1850s. MacIntyre (1984) contended that such changes are part and parcel of the nature of a practice. Accordingly, changes in the technical skills used in nursing would not necessarily change the inherent nature of nursing as a practice. Further, MacIntyre (1984) contended that in a practice, "the relevant goods and ends which the technical skills serve—and every practice does require the exercise of technical skills—are transformed and enriched by . . . extensions of human powers" (p. 193). Nursing, as a practice, may extend the good toward which it is aimed by disclosing and realizing the possibilities inherent within it. According to MacIntyre, this is necessary if a practice is to remain alive. But what good are we talking about when it comes to the practice of nursing?

In descriptions of nursing since the mid-20th century, it is difficult to discern the good sought because nursing has been defined merely in terms of a list of activities or as an art and a science. Descriptions of nursing have also focused on nursing as a profession and whether it is indeed a profession. The lack of specification of the good toward which nursing practice is aimed could be a result of the fact that in much of early nursing research, the empirical methods of the sciences were used more out of a desire to establish nursing as a discipline within the academic community than out of a desire to foster the well-being of patients. However, in the past decade, nursing scholars have begun to focus on articulating the essence of nursing from the perspective of the practice itself. Patricia Benner (1984) thoroughly described the domains and competencies of nursing practice in a manner that recognizes the diversity and complexity of nursing practice. Through them, she articulated what the good is in nursing. Although she did not articulate what she perceived to be the moral sense of nursing, it is evident from the exemplars of excellence she cited that nurses do have a moral sense.

THE MORAL SENSE OF NURSING

John Scudder and I (Bishop & Scudder, 1990, 1991) articulated the moral sense of nursing in terms of fostering the well-being of patients. We arrived at this moral sense of nursing from a study of 40 nurses who described their most fulfilling experiences as nurses. All of the descriptions, except one, spoke to either the moral or the personal sources of fulfillment. The one exception was a nurse whom I had to interview to determine whether her fulfillment came from the moral, personal, professional, or technical aspects of nursing. When she was finally forced to choose, she said that in the particular story that she had related, her fulfillment had come from the technical. However, she also stated she would not stay in nursing if the technical was all there was to nursing.

Brenda's story makes evident the moral sense of nursing. It is clear from her story that she was concerned for JoAnn's well-being. Similarly, the exemplars in Benner's (1984) study demonstrate that most nurses are very concerned about fostering the well-being of their patients. The aim of fostering patient well-being is also expressed by students entering nursing school, who say that they entered nursing because they wanted to help others.

Young students wanting to help others, the stories in Benner's (1984) study, and other nurses' stories, such as Brenda's, have in common not only a moral sense of nursing but also a focus on relationships of nurses and patients as relationships of human being to human being. It is in this connectedness of human beings that we can find the third essential of nursing—caring.

NURSING AS A PRACTICE OF CARING

Carol Gilligan (1982) studied the ways in which women make moral decisions and found that they make them quite differently from men. She stated, "To admit the truth of the women's perspective to the conception of moral development is to recognize for both sexes the importance throughout life of the connection between self and other, the universality of the need for compassion and care" (p. 98). The work of nursing necessarily involves compassion and care. However, in speaking of what nurses do, it is often said that nurses give nursing care rather than that they care, not only in the sense of an activity but also in the sense of concern for others.

It is only recently that nursing scholars have attempted to interpret the meaning of *care* and *caring*. To interpret *caring* merely as giving care to a patient or as a subjective feeling of beneficence toward another person is to limit the significance of caring, especially in a profession such as nursing. Gilligan (1982) contended that "the ideal of care is thus an activity of relationship, of seeing, and responding to need, taking care of the world by sustaining the web of connection so that no one is left alone" (p. 62). It is in this web of connection that nurses care.

Nell Noddings (1984) further extended our understanding of caring when she described the essential elements in a caring relationship as "*engrossment* and *motivational displacement* on the part of the one-caring and a form of *responsiveness* or *reciprocity* on the part of the cared-for" (p. 150). Brenda does not tell us very much about her initial encounter with JoAnn the night she first came to the clinic. However, we do know that even though JoAnn had no specific complaints, Brenda took her seriously and ordered some diagnostic laboratory work. Brenda wondered later about what might have happened if she had not called JoAnn immediately—if she had become involved with something else. I believe her action exemplifies what Noddings called a motivational shift, a "motive energy [that] flows toward the other" (p. 33). The responsiveness and reciprocity on the part of the cared-for can be seen in JoAnn's following of Brenda's instruction to go to the emergency room immediately. Her reciprocity is also reflected in her return to the clinic and in her thanking Brenda for possibly having saved her life.

In her discussion of caring, Noddings (1984) also distinguished between natural caring and ethical caring. According to Noddings, natural caring comes from a remembrance of being cared for, whereas ethical caring "is an active relation between my actual self and a vision of my ideal self as one-caring and cared-for" (p. 49). In other words, nurses may care naturally or they may care out of the desire to be a good nurse. When nurses care, whether naturally or ethically, they live the moral sense of nursing. Nurses have a moral obligation to act on behalf of patients or clients in a manner that fosters their healing and health. Patients' health is fostered by nursing care whether they are recovering from open heart surgery; are new mothers with healthy infants; are taking a class at a nursing center on how to control blood pressure; or need clean surroundings, good diet, and fresh air to heal. The hospital nurse, the community health nurse, and the nurse educator are all focused on fostering the physical and psychological health and well-being of the other.

Conclusion

Is nursing conventional in the sense that its meaning requires historical interpretation to determine its evolving nature, or does nursing have an essence with an ahistorical meaning? In some ways, nursing today looks like the nursing of Nightingale's day; in other ways, it is quite different. What nurses "do," in terms of technical skills, whether in hospitals or in home health, has changed dramatically from Nightingale's time and even during the time that I have been in nursing. However, the changes in nursing skills and competencies that become apparent when we look at nursing over time are clearly a part of the essence of nursing that can be found when we go to "the things themselves"—nursing practice. When we examine nursing itself, we find that it is inherently a caring practice with a moral sense. The moral sense of nursing is the commitment of nursing to foster the healing and health of people that it serves. This moral sense in itself necessitates that nursing change as new ways of healing and fostering health become known. This moral commitment focuses on the charge to care—to care naturally if we can and, if we cannot care naturally, then to care ethically because we want to be good nurses.

For me, the important problem is not whether the nature of nursing is natural or conventional, but whether we, as nurses, consider the nature of nursing and whether, having considered it, we can articulate it in a way that recognizes the complexities of the practice without losing sight of our primary moral purpose as nurses.

References

American Nurses' Association. (1980). *Nursing: A social policy statement*. Kansas City, MO: Author.

Benner, P. (1984). *From novice to expert: Excellence and power in clinical nursing practice*. Menlo Park, CA: Addison-Wesley.

Bishop, A., & Scudder, J. R., Jr. (1990). *The practical, moral, and personal sense of nursing: A phenomenological philosophy of practice.* Albany: State University of New York Press.

Bishop, A., & Scudder, J. R., Jr. (1991). *Nursing: The practice of caring.* New York: National League for Nursing.

Gilligan, C. (1982). *In a different voice: Psychological theory and women's moral development.* Cambridge, MA: Harvard University Press.

Heidegger, M. (1962). *Being and time* (J. Macquarrie & E. Robinson, Trans.). New York: Harper & Row.

Husserl, E. (1965). *Phenomenology and the crisis of philosophy* (Q. Lauer, Trans.). New York: Harper & Row. (Original work published 1911)

MacIntyre, A. (1984). *After virtue* (2nd ed.). Notre Dame, IN: University of Notre Dame Press.

Nightingale, F. (1946). *Notes on nursing: What it is and what it is not.* Philadelphia: J. B. Lippincott. (Original work published 1859)

Noddings, N. (1984). *Caring: A feminine approach to ethics and moral education.* Berkeley: University of California Press.

Ricoeur, P. (1977). Phenomenology and the social sciences. In M. Korenbaum (Ed.), *Annals of Phenomenological Sociology II* (pp. 145-159). Dayton, OH: Wright State University.

CHAPTER 8

Common Sense, Truth, and Nursing Knowledge Development

ROZELLA M. SCHLOTFELDT

Disciplinary knowledge development is generally considered to be a responsibility of scholars who are competent to engage in systematic inquiry. They do so by identifying gaps in existing knowledge, discrediting knowledge known to be outdated or in error, and discovering new knowledge—all of which can be depended on to keep disciplinary knowledge current.

Scholars in the recognized professions, like those in the basic disciplines, similarly and typically hold responsibility for discovering knowledge that is unique to their respective professions and that makes up a major portion of their profession's body of knowledge. In addition, some scholars in the professions, who are deemed to be so qualified, hold responsibility for selecting and incorporating into the body of knowledge of their profession verified truths from relevant disciplines that are essential to the practice of their profession. For example, whereas physician-scholars are responsible for discovering knowledge that is unique to the medical profession, physician-scholars who are also geneticists must be depended on to select and incorporate into the body of medical knowledge verified genetic knowledge of causative factors in human pathologies.

The knowledge that has been agreed upon by designated scholars within each profession at any particular time in history constitutes that profession's body of knowledge and defines it. It is in fact the intellectual armamentarium that students of the profession must master, internalize, and use creatively, ethically, and effectively in fulfilling the profession's institutionalized social goal or mission within the society its practitioners serve.

This chapter addresses the role of common sense in arriving at truths that are fundamental to the sustained development of nursing knowledge. That knowledge is essential to nursing's progress toward becoming recognized as a primary health profession and as a scholarly academic discipline. What, then, is the appropriate contribution of common sense to truth and to nursing knowledge development? First, some definitions are necessary.

Definitions

Common sense is defined in the *American Heritage Dictionary* (1985) as "native good judgment . . . that is shared by the community as a whole" (pp. 298-299). And, in that same dictionary, *truth* is defined as being "in accordance with reality" (p. 1300). The latter definition must surely have been based upon the conviction that truths about reality can be established through systematic inquiry of several kinds and through commonsense reasoning. Commonsense judgment is what armchair philosophers use to test the validity of the conclusions that emerge from philosophical inquiry concerning the existence of everything in light of what is called "first causes" (Adler, 1965, pp. 79-80).

It is the thesis of this chapter that truths about the nature of human beings in relation to their health can be derived from common sense, from thoughtful observation and consideration of the experiences common to nurses and to other persons. In addition, truths about the nature of nursing, as an existing, beneficially consequential service to human beings that deserves recognition as a health care discipline and profession, can be so established. Both truths about the nature of human beings and truths about the nature of nursing are essential to the development of nursing knowledge.

The Nature of Human Beings

There is probably no field of work comparable to nursing that offers its practitioners as many opportunities to enter into experiences from which they can draw commonsense conclusions concerning the nature of human beings as it relates to their health and health care. Consider, for example, the wonder of thoughtful students of nursing who, for the first time, encounter newly born infants, even those prematurely born. Those nursing students must surely be stimulated by this experience to think deeply about the magnificent native endowment of these infants, who demonstrate the ability and the propensity to seek and obtain nutrition, to exercise and develop their muscles, to move around sufficiently to attain comfort, and to communicate their discomfort and need for attention.

With rare exception, though infirm and thus dependent at birth, human infants are endowed with physical, physiological, intellectual, and psychological mechanisms and manifest social behaviors that can logically be called native health-seeking assets essential to their sustained growth and development. Given a caring and enlightened environment and needed resources, infants develop and demonstrate the interest, ability, will, and determination gradually to reject the dependency that accompanied their immaturity and to attain increasing independence in executing their own programs of health care.

The multiple and varied clinical experiences of nursing students and all nursing practitioners allow them to conclude, on the basis of their common sense, that in circumstances of relative health, injury, and illness, children, youths, adults, and the elderly value and seek to attain, retain, and regain optimal health and to become and remain independent in executing their own programs of health care as they know and understand them. Parents, teachers, and other careful observers of human beings surely must join nurses in the commonsense conclusion that humans are by nature health-seeking beings. Further, they know that health is a variable concept.

The dictionary definition of *health* is "soundness, especially of body and mind [and] freedom from disease or abnormality" (*American Heritage Dictionary*, 1985, p. 599). Although this definition is widely accepted as reasonable, everyone knows that there are human beings who are afflicted with chronic diseases and disabilities and who are, from their own perspective, "healthy." They are able to lead normal, productive, and satisfying lives because of their compensatory abilities and because their disease pathologies are reasonably well controlled. In considering such individuals, common sense reveals that it is the individual's place on the independence-dependence continuum that determines his or her need for nursing care.

What, then, is the nature of nursing, and what is the role of common sense in arriving at truths about the nature of nursing?

The Nature of Nursing

Nursing has been in existence for almost one and a half centuries. Beginning in the mid-1800s, Florence Nightingale, a brilliant, advantaged, and well-educated woman, demonstrated that nursing is a beneficially consequential human service by preparing women to provide the care needed by the ill, wounded, and dying soldiers of England's army during the Crimean War (Nutting & Dock, 1909, pp. 117-171). This dramatic demonstration encouraged Nightingale's supporters to provide her with the opportunity to establish a school of nursing at St. Thomas Hospital in London. Here she demonstrated the effectiveness of a new educational system for nurses and thereby established a new field of work for women (Nutting & Dock, 1909, pp. 172-206).

In 1859, Nightingale recorded her cogent observations in a published treatise entitled *Notes on Nursing*. In that classic volume, she noted that nursing's goal and practice domain are "to put the patient in the best condition for nature to act on him" (1859/1965, p. 75). She thereby gave recognition to human beings' native abilities and propensities to seek and attain health. She further noted that "nature's laws of health or of nursing . . . are in reality the same" (p. 6). In stating that those laws were, at the time, unknown, Nightingale foresaw the need for nursing knowledge development and nursing's research agenda.

Nursing and preservice nursing education were established in North America initially in 1873, according to Nightingale's plan (Stewart, 1943, pp. 83-119). They flourished across Canada and the United States as hospitals multiplied to accommodate the recognized medical and health care needs of a westward migrating population.

During the first half of the twentieth century, nursing leaders in North America devoted their time and energy to improving the quality of preservice preparation of nurses and to obtaining legal status for nurses through nurse registration procedures. This latter goal began to be realized early in the decade as nurse registration gradually became a reality. The former goal, to improve the quality of preservice preparation of nurses, was set as a result of several studies that demonstrated major defects in the education of nursing students (Stewart, 1943, pp. 187-238). The solution, according to some nursing leaders, was to seek and secure relationships with universities whose faculties would teach nursing students the science (and, later, the humanities) content that, in their view, nursing students should know. Affiliation agreements with universities were developed by hospital school officials, and some universities began to accept nursing schools as autonomous units within their institutions. In the university-controlled nursing programs, typically, university professors determined the content of the science and humanities courses, and physicians taught nursing students content related to human pathologies and diagnostic and treatment modalities that they thought nurses should know. Nursing principles and practices were taught by nursing faculty.

During this same time period, questions concerning the nature of nursing were answered by the conducting of task analysis studies designed to identify what nurses were doing at that time (Jameson & Sewall, 1954, p. 440). Nurses, however, in response to recommendations that nurses should control nursing and nursing education, continued to write textbooks that set forth the principles that rationalized nursing practices. Henderson (1960) was one such author who, over several years, revised her texts and her definition of nursing that conveyed her conceptualization of nursing.

In 1960, Henderson's definition of nursing was given worldwide sanction by virtue of its acceptance by all of the nursing organizations that were then members of the International Council of Nurses (Henderson, 1960). Her definition of nursing surely reflects common-sense truths about human beings and nursing (as previously noted here). It explicates nursing's essential goal and social mission as follows:

> The unique function of the nurse is to assist the individual, sick or well, in the performance of those activities contributing to health or its recovery (or to a peaceful death) that he would perform unaided if he had the necessary strength, will or knowledge. And to do this in such a way as to help him gain independence as rapidly as possible. (p. 3)

In contrast to these beliefs about the nature of nursing, in 1980, the American Nurses' Association (ANA) published its *Social Policy Statement,* in which nursing's traditional roles and definitions were rejected and replaced by a definition that, though claiming to "maintain [nursing's] historical orientation" (p. 9) toward the promotion of human health, was in fact oriented to the diagnosis and treatment of health problems. The ANA defined *nursing* as "the diagnosis and treatment of human responses to actual or potential health problems" (p. 9). A detailed critique of that definition appears elsewhere (Schlotfeldt, 1987). Certainly, a more accurate definition of nursing could be derived from thoughtful observations of truly professional nurses providing care to persons who are essentially well and to those who, as a result of mild or serious illness, are in relative states of dependence as a consequence of their inadequate knowledge, skill, strength, and will. The definition must also heed the dying patient. Such a commonsense definition of nursing is here proposed:

> Nursing is the appraisal and the enhancement of the health status, health-seeking assets, and health potentials of human beings during their

relative dependence with regard to their health care and assisting them to attain independence while preserving their human dignity during their dependent states and at the time of death.

Undoubtedly, that definition could be improved upon. However, it does reflect commonsense conclusions about the nature of human beings and the nature of nursing as it has traditionally existed for more than a century, as it exists now, and as it is likely to exist in the future.

Nursing Knowledge Development

Several major events influenced nurses' orientation to their work and scholarly endeavors. By the early 1950s, leaders within nursing began to emphasize nurses' responsibility as investigators to select, discover, and organize the knowledge basic to nursing practice. However, because there were few nurses qualified to prepare future nurse investigators and because science was considered to be the preferred route to scholarship and verified knowledge, most nurse scholars chose doctoral study in the sciences. A few studied philosophy with a view toward identifying the moral and ethical bases of nursing practice. Others had already become prepared as educators, administrators, and historians.

By the late 1960s and 1970s, doctoral programs in nursing were developed and thereafter became the preferred preparation for scholars in nursing. Nursing leaders called for conceptualizations of nursing that reflected the perspective of nursing and its values. Subsequently, several such conceptualizations reflective of the philosophic orientation of their authors were developed and became guides for nursing practice, education, and research. The authors of those conceptualizations were considered to be theorists, but their conceptualizations were not generally recognized as philosophical in nature. Despite the establishment of doctoral programs in nursing, science continued to be valued as the road to truth, undoubtedly reflecting the scientific preparation that most of nursing's scholars had received during their doctoral study in the sciences. Upon completing such study and returning to nursing faculties, nursing's scientists developed research programs that reflected their scientific orientation.

The urgent need now is for an official nursing organization made up of qualified scholars, including nursing historians, philosophers, scientists, and practicing clinicians, to come to agreement about the nature of nursing's body of knowledge. It is imperative that the body of nursing knowledge include knowledge of nursing's heritage: first as an existing craft; then as a vocation and later as a technology; and now, at least in part, as a profession with the potential to become a learned profession. The body of nursing knowledge will have to be continuously under development and updated and to include knowledge of means to identify and measure human health status, health potentials, and health-seeking assets (i.e., human beings' native and acquired health-seeking mechanisms and behaviors). Also necessary for inclusion will be knowledge of factors that influence human health and knowledge that informs nursing's strategies (e.g., strategies of appraisal, compensation, guiding and supporting, teaching, stimulating, and even inspiring, as well as means to determine their relative efficacy in assisting human beings achieve independence in executing appropriate health care regimes).

Conclusion

When common sense is utilized to reach agreement regarding the nature of human beings, of nursing, and of nursing knowledge and when means for the continuous development and updating of nursing's body of knowledge are established, nursing will finally become the recognized profession that its members have so long expected it to become. Furthermore, nursing knowledge will become recognized as the academic discipline it so richly deserves to be.

References

Adler, M. J. (1965). *The conditions of philosophy*. New York: Atheneum.
American Heritage Dictionary (2nd ed.). (1985). Boston: Houghton Mifflin.

American Nurses' Association. (1980). *Nursing: A social policy statement*. Kansas City, MO: Author.

Henderson, V. (1960). *Basic principles of nursing care*. London: International Council of Nurses.

Jameson, E., & Sewall, M. (1954). *Trends in nursing history* (4th ed.). Philadelphia: W. B. Saunders.

Nightingale, F. (1965). *Notes on nursing: What it is and what it is not*. Philadelphia: University of Pennsylvania Press. (Original work published 1859)

Nutting, M., & Dock, L. (1909). *A history of nursing* (Vol. 2). New York: Putnam's Sons.

Schlotfeldt, R. (1987). Defining nursing: A historic controversy. *Nursing Research, 36*, 64-67.

Stewart, I. (1943). *The education of nurses*. New York: Macmillan.

PART III

Expressions of Truth in Nursing Inquiry

It is one thing to have grasped a truth; it is quite another to communicate it. This Plato realized. In *The Republic,* Plato (1928) resorted to myths to capture and convey the meaning of complex ideas (e.g., the Form of the good) when he found that he could not do so adequately using the abstract prose of philosophy. Plato was of the mind that not all that one knows can be put forward in declarative form (Jones, 1976). Similarly, a growing number of nurse scholars, finding the language and methods of traditional science wanting in terms of capturing and conveying nursing truths, have begun to look for other ways of doing so.

In the essays contained in Part III of this volume, newly emerging ways of expressing truth in nursing inquiry are described. In Chapter 9, Sandelowski discusses storytelling in nursing inquiry, identifying similarities between theory and story construction. In Chapter 10, Watson describes how, in poetic form, truth can be conveyed in nursing inquiry. Given that nursing is an art and that storytelling and poetry lie within the realm of art, these new-found ways appear to be more akin to nursing than those that lie in the realm of science (traditional science). But the question remains: Are the newly emerging ways of expressing truth appropriate to nursing inquiry? In Chapter 11, Romyn takes up this question in relation to the epistemological and methodological underpinnings of feminist research.

This matter of appropriateness ought to be taken up before *any* new method of inquiry is seriously adopted. That said, how is appropriateness of method to be determined? It would seem that whether a particular method of attaining or expressing nursing truth is appropriate depends on what ought to be sought in nursing inquiry—that is, on its aim. For example, if we agree with nurse scholars such as Schlotfeldt (1988) that an organized body of nursing knowledge is the aim of our research, then we will evaluate a particular method in terms of its adequacy as a means to this end. It goes without saying that this evaluation will entail a consideration of the method's potential to contribute to the attainment of nursing's unique object. This is so because a discipline develops a body of organized knowledge of its own only for the sake of attaining its object.

Considering the adequacy of a particular method in terms of the object of nursing poses a problem, however, because to date there has been little agreement on what nursing's object is. Given the diversity of entities (e.g., caring, health, and human becoming) that have been taken to be nursing's object and the multitude of ways in which each has been conceived, a particular method may be judged to be appropriate and adequate under one object or conception but not under another. The consequence for the development of an organized body of nursing knowledge is devastatingly clear.

References

Jones, W. T. (1976). *A history of Western philosophy: Vol. 1. The classical mind* (2nd ed.). New York: Harcourt Brace Jovanovich.

Plato. (1928). *The Republic.* New York: Scribner.

Schlotfeldt, R. M. (1988). Structuring nursing knowledge: A priority for creating nursing's future. *Nursing Science Quarterly, 1*(1), 35-38.

Guiding Questions:
Making up Your Own Mind

Can all nursing truths be communicated in propositional form? If not, would those truths that cannot be so communicated be found in nursing's body of knowledge?

What is the relationship between the meaningful, the useful, and the truthful?

Are narratives and poetry means of expressing truth in all sciences or only in nursing science?

Are narratives and poetry expressive of either speculative or practical nursing truth?

What do narratives and poetry as expressions of truth have in common?

If poetical truth characterizes the fine arts and if nursing pursues poetical truth, can one conclude that nursing is one of the fine arts? If so, would nursing then no longer seek logical or factual truth in that fine arts do not?

If poetical truth, as opposed to logical or factual truth, is taken to be the goal of nursing inquiry, what would that imply for nursing practice?

What, if anything, differentiates storytelling in nursing science, storytelling in nursing history, and storytelling in fiction?

What is the goal of nursing inquiry—knowledge, power, or something else?

In nursing inquiry, are all expressions of truth gender specific? context specific? relationship specific?

In context-specific inquiry, are there any necessary limits on the extension or breadth of the context?

CHAPTER 9

Truth/Storytelling
in Nursing Inquiry

MARGARETE J. SANDELOWSKI

*When talking about their lives, people lie sometimes, forget a lot,
exaggerate, become confused, and get things wrong. Yet they are
revealing truths. These truths don't reveal the past "as it actually
was," aspiring to a standard of objectivity. They give us instead the
truths of our experiences. They aren't the result of empirical
research or the logic of mathematical deductions. Unlike the
reassuring Truth of the scientific ideal, the truths of personal
narratives are neither open to proof nor self-evident. We come to
understand them only through interpretation, paying careful
attention to the contexts that shape their creation and to the world
views that inform them. (Personal Narratives Group, 1989, p. 261)*

This is a chapter about telling stories, telling truths, and the continui-
ties between them. In it, I emphasize the similarities between entities

that we have typically been taught to think of as different from and even as opposed to each other. By choosing to emphasize their similarities, I neither deny their differences nor assume the superiority of one over the other by virtue of these differences.

Most of us have been taught in our theory and methods courses to see science and story, and truth and fiction, from an "either/or" perspective. We have learned to glorify and even anxiously to strive toward the factors on the left of each of these supposedly oppositional pairs—science and truth. At the same time, we have learned also to disparage the factors on the right—story and fiction, "ferociously . . . distanc[ing]" (Hunter, 1990, p. 8) ourselves from anything that could be construed as unscientific and therefore untrue. We have been taught that our goal in conducting research is to get the truth, the whole truth, and nothing but the truth. Assured that this goal is attainable, we have been enjoined to master the techniques with which to defend the truth from those ever-present threats (of which we have also been repeatedly warned) to the internal and external validity of our projects.

Yet, as I argue in this chapter, we might better serve the human subjects of our research by conceiving the goal of inquiry as getting, not the whole truth, but rather the *whole story*. Moreover, we might better serve ourselves as inquirers by recognizing that our conventional notion of truth itself constitutes one of our most cherished "cultural stories" (Richardson, 1990a, p. 127). Cultural stories are moral and cautionary tales told from the point of view of the normative order that serves to maintain the status quo. Such stories, by *seeming true,* maintain their hold on the imagination of the members of the culture that created them.

The Trouble With Truth

Underlying the almost evangelical and somewhat militaristic conception of science and truth that I have just described are the assumptions that only science is concerned with truth; there is a one-and-only Truth out there waiting to be discovered; and that a valid study, finding, or conclusion is true. The "trouble with truth" (Goodman, 1978, p. 17) as we have typically conceived it is that scientists cannot exclusively claim it. Artists, for example, also seek the truth and often produce works of art that are more *true to life* than either science or even life itself. Indeed, artists often illuminate the human condition by avoiding the so-called *whole truth* through eliminating trivial, transient, and other particular elements that might impede the comprehension of some essential feature of human nature (Hospers, 1946). As Nisbet (1976) observed, "A tragedy or comedy is, after all, no less an inquiry into reality, no less a distillation of perceptions and experiences, than a hypothesis or theory that undertakes to account for the variable incidence of murder or marriage" (p. 12). Even wildly fanciful departures from camera truth in paintings may be in the service of fidelity to the subject matter (Hospers, 1946).

Moreover, truth is plural as opposed to singular; truths are social products "of the moment" (Rosenwald, 1988, p. 259) and of different "worlds" (Bruner, 1986; Goodman, 1978). As Goodman (1978) stated, truth can be neither defined nor tested by agreement with *the* world because truths differ for different worlds. In addition, the nature of agreement between any "version" of the world and the world itself is "notoriously nebulous" and is taken to be true only so long as it "offends no unyielding beliefs and none of its own precepts" (p. 17). Furthermore, the goal of determining "the truth, the whole truth, and nothing but the truth" is, at the least, perverse and, at the most, paralyzing. The whole truth would be too much, and nothing but the truth would be too little (Goodman, 1978, p. 19).

The trouble with validity, as we have typically conceived it, is that it is thought to be equivalent to or synonymous with truth. It is not: The premises and conclusions of a valid argument can be false (Goodman, 1978, p. 125). Also, two independent measures of a phenomenon may both be invalid as measures of that phenomenon and may therefore seriously compromise the goal of criterion-related validity (Deutscher, 1970). Moreover, techniques employed to ensure validity typically produce findings that are in turn validated by those techniques; the rules for playing the game of research are also the criteria for evaluating the product of research (Morgan, 1983).

A more valid notion of validity, in terms of correspondence to the actual everyday work of scientists, is that it is the end product of a social process of validation in which the truth claims made for a project may be either accepted or rejected by a community of scholars. Whether qualitative researchers or "experimentalists," we all depend for the validation of our projects on "contextually grounded linguistic and interpretive practices" (Mishler, 1990, p. 421) characteristic of a particular research tradition. Validity is therefore neither an absolute nor a universal entity corresponding to one truth. Accordingly, the problem of validity is not resolved simply by adherence to standardized technical solutions to minimize threats to validity.

By admitting the socially constructed nature of truth, we are able to treat it not as a "solemn and severe master," but rather as a "docile and obedient servant" (Goodman, 1978, p. 18). Scientists, no less than other truth seekers, tailor their truths to fit a prevailing sense of how things are or ought to be. They, no less than other explorers and creators, *decree* the scientific laws they discover and *design* the patterns in nature they discern. Both theoretical and narrative accounts are co-created and recreated in every interaction between observer and nature or listener and teller. Indeed, when we conceive of truth as the fixed and acontextual—ahistorical, abiographical, and acultural—product of a singular kind of quest, we deceive ourselves. More important, when we emphasize the difference between truth telling in science and truth telling in stories and the superiority of the former over the latter, we serve only to retell one of our most cherished cultural stories: the one in which science is portrayed as completely unlike, superior to, and always triumphing over story.

A Theory of Story

Although we are inclined to see them as wholly different entities, scientific theories and the everyday stories that we often hear in qualitative interviews have many things in common. Indeed, as I noted in a previous paper on the topic of the narrative (Sandelowski, 1991), some scholars have argued that all science begins with stories and that scientific theories are themselves a kind of story. Like theories, stories are renderings of events made up and re-presented by human beings. They are, therefore, "no more fictional than any other product of thought" (Robinson & Hawpe, 1986, p. 111). Like theories, stories are means to interpret events: to "construct a causal pattern" that integrates what is known and conjectured about an event (Robinson & Hawpe, 1986, p. 112). A story, no less than a theory, is, therefore, a "candidate for veracity, subject to challenge by others" who might have a better theory or story (Gergen & Gergen, 1988, p. 31). Theory making, no less than story making, involves the use of rhetorical devices and techniques to "quiet our initial objections to their unreality" (Tirrell, 1990, p. 124).

Indeed, both theories and stories have to meet certain criteria and even some of the same criteria to be evaluated as good. Both theories and stories are typically judged to be *good* when they are believable, coherent, consistent, and intelligible; good theories and good stories provide a sense of understanding, order, and aesthetic finality.

To meet the criterion of believability, for example, both a theory and a story must offer a good "fit" with experience and/or a "coherent and plausible account of how and why something happened" (Robinson & Hawpe, 1986, p. 111). In both theory and story, this involves the selection and selective (re)arrangement of facts or events that will yield the most satisfying and even pleasing account. Krieger (1991) suggested that social science is, in effect, a self-comforting activity whereby scientists make up stories to fit the world. Moreover, when confronted with the choice between truth and beauty, scientists, like (other) storytellers, will often choose beauty (Chandrasekhar, 1987). As Hunter (1990) observed, "In the rhetoric of science, facts may be irrefutable, but beauty is compelling" (p. 7). To a scientist, for example, parsimony is beautiful; "A parsimonious theory is one that is *elegant* [italics added] in its simplicity even though it may be broad in its content" (Walker & Avant, 1988, p. 147). Scientists often favor the elegant simplicity of generalities to the tedious precision of particulars. Indeed, "generalizations always tell a little lie in the service of (what is considered by scientists to be) a greater truth" (Earley, 1988, p. 205).

To meet the criterion of intelligibility, both a theory and a story must be understandable and recognizable *as a theory or story* to their respective audiences. Both theorist and storyteller must abide by culturally acceptable (as defined by one's ethnic group or discipline) rules of theory and story construction. Indeed, because the construction of both theories and stories is not so much fact driven (with facts themselves theory laden) as it is governed by conventions for their construction (Gergen & Gergen, 1988), truth telling in theory or story is *limited by the rules for telling the truth* in each of these forms.[1] Walker and Avant's (1988) popular text on theory construction in nursing, for example, is an excellent illustration of the conventions of this genre of representing reality.

A storied description or explanation of events, no less than a theoretical one, must conform to the conventions of story making to be accepted. Gergen and Gergen (1986, 1988) proposed that there are only three primitive narrative forms available for rendering life events: (a) the progressive, or happily-ever-after, narrative, in which events are arranged to indicate movement toward a desired goal; (b) the regressive, or tragic, narrative, in which events are arranged to indicate movement away from a goal; and (c) the stability narrative, in which no movement is indicated. Narrators use combinations of these forms, as in the regressive to progressive (comedic/melodramatic) narrative and in the alternatively regressive and progressive (romantic) narrative.

Cultural conventions for theory or story construction may make these forms unrecognizable and therefore unintelligible to those unfamiliar with these conventions. For example, in her account of the difficulty experienced by an Anglo-American interviewer in understanding a Puerto Rican narrator's account of the dissolution of her marriage, Riessman (1987) demonstrated that a story organized episodically, as opposed to temporally, may not be grasped by a listener expecting and "intuitively understanding" a temporally ordered narrative (p. 176). Gergen and Gergen (1986, 1988) described the typical Western story as one that is organized temporally (but not necessarily in clock time), with events selected for their relevance to a goal state and falling on an evaluative continuum in relation to some end point.

In a related vein, the entire notion of "member validation" (Bloor, 1983) as a means to ensure the credibility of our interpretations of qualitative data may be undermined by scholarly conventions for re-presenting them. For example, an adoptive mother in my study of infertile couples' transition to parenthood conveyed to me her difficulty in understanding my account, which I had written for an academic publication, of the experiences of adopting couples that included her account. What caused her difficulty was not that my account was untrue, but rather the way I chose to render the findings. As researchers and academicians, we typically choose to re-present research participants' stories in ways that will be recognized, not by the original narrators as their stories, but rather by other researchers as good science. Accordingly, member validation may have ethical and rhetorical dimensions yet to be recognized; we may give our findings to narrators to evaluate in a form they will recognize, but that may well be very different from the form in which their stories are offered to the academic public.

Not only does the criterion of intelligibility mandate that truths be disseminated or "encoded" in different forms for different audiences (Richardson, 1990b, p. 32), but it may also demand foregoing a truth in its favor. For example, a linear or actual clock-time accounting of events may not be the most effective means to achieve intelligibility (Gergen & Gergen, 1988; Riessman, 1987). This point was brought home to me in one infertile woman's account of how she finally came to be pregnant. This woman, another participant in one of my studies of infertility, found it important to interrupt her sequential accounting of the events that occurred related to her infertility with what she called "a side story" of her successful self-treatment of a chronic illness that preceded her infertility. She assured me that I would find this narrative detour "significant in the long run" in understanding her triumph over infertility. She was right; she used this story strategically (Riessman, 1990) to cast herself as a woman able to counter conventional medical therapies successfully and to represent infertility as yet another occasion demanding that she "fight for myself" against great odds.

Importantly, the narrative sequence of events in her story did not correspond to the actual sequence of events in her life, but this very lack of correspondence made her story better and more true to her experience. She told the *whole story,* even if not, by virtue of its lack of correspondence to the sequencing of actual events, the *whole truth.* Her narrative illustrates well how strict adherence to a one-to-one correspondence (to empirical reality) view of truth may actually take us further away from the truth. Also, her story foregrounds a circumstance in which the whole truth was appropriately sacrificed to intelligibility in the service of telling the whole story that was *truer to life.* Similar sacrifices are made in scientific theory construction in the service of meeting such criteria as intelligibility, utility, and parsimony.

Although conventions can be and are resisted, this resistance is often achieved at the price of intelligibility and believability. Consider, for example, Gergen and Gergen's (1988) observation that the typical North American story of old age is a regressive narrative of decline and disability, whereas the typical Asian story is a progressive narrative of maturity, wisdom, and honor. Accordingly, North Americans will tend not to question a regressive account of old age but may, at the very least, suspend their belief in a progressive account: Such an account will not ring true to them. As a related point, Gergen (1988) argued that people's renderings of events or developmental periods in their lives conform as much to prevailing cultural stories about these events and periods as to their actual experiences of them. In other words, an individual's account of what "was" often includes or is a version of what "must have been" (p. 107).

Of importance, too, is that different (ethnic and disciplinary) cultures "invite" (Gergen & Gergen, 1988, p. 28) different stories and therefore different expectations of those stories from audiences, which may either accept or reject them as stories. The "ontological security" of both storyteller and theorist is, accordingly, in the "public domain" (Gergen & Gergen, 1988, p. 40): Both are equally dependent on accounts that are acceptable to their respective publics. In the sense that stories are accepted as good/true only if certain conventions are observed, narrative construction is no more free of constraints than theory construction. Indeed, whether a given story or theory is deemed valid depends at least as much (and, some argue, more) on observing these conventions than on any absolute correspondence between a rendering of an event and the event itself.

Interestingly, consistency seems to be a more important criterion for both theory and story construction than correspondence to some empirical reality. Yet even consistency may be sacrificed in storytelling as narrators try out different explanations of an event, often within the confines of a single interview (Blaxter, 1983). I observed this lack of consistency in couples' explanations of their infertility within the same interview and between interviews with the same couples over time (Sandelowski, Holditch-Davis, & Harris, 1990). Indeed, it was the analytic problem that this observation presented that ultimately led me to scholarship in the area of narrative.

As I read about the nature of storytelling, I came to understand that the lack of consistency I had observed was evidence not of the couples' unreliability as informants, but rather of the constant revisionist nature of narratives—each telling is a retelling. In a "remembering moment" (Spence, 1982, p. 3), the couples struggled to achieve the most internally consistent interpretation of the past-in-the-present, the experienced present, and the anticipated-in-the-present future.

Stories, therefore, may not have the "diachronic" or "synchronic" reliability (Kirk & Miller, 1986, p. 42) we typically seek to support validity claims. The assumption (operationalized in test-retest measures) that a configuration of data should be isomorphic over time denies history and change. Further, the assumption that similarity of observations concerning a target event should be achieved at a single time (operationalized in split-half measures) may result in failure to address how different observations might simultaneously be true.

Finally, like a good theory, a good story has elements of universality. In what Rosenwald (1988) described as the "doctrinal riot" between those celebrating abstractness and generalizability and those celebrating concreteness and particularity (p. 240), we have ignored the idea of individual lives and life stories as mutually relevant to, and even in conversation with, each other. Lives are lived and told in context (Watson, 1976, 1989). Because individuals live and narrate their lives in time and place, they provide us with knowledge about much more than themselves. Indeed, Gergen and Gergen (1988) argued that narratives of the self are not "fundamentally possessions of the individual" at all, but rather products of "social interchange" (p. 18).

Although we may not always recognize it, we see ourselves and others as part of, and in or out of synchrony with, history and culture. When several of the married couples in my study described themselves to me as "late" getting married or "late" having a child, they were telling me something about themselves and about cultural norms that specify when individuals may think of themselves as being on time or off time, normal or deviant. When one woman unable to have biological children made a point of describing herself to me as not bothered by this inability "like other women," she was comparing herself to other infertile women and both reminding me of and resisting the cultural story of infertility in which infertility is typically emplotted as a biological and emotional disability for women. When an adoptive father of an Asian baby described to me how he and his wife came to view biology as unimportant to the establishment of the parent-child bond, he was not only telling me the particulars of this revelation for him and his wife but also foregrounding the primacy of the blood tie between parent and child, characteristic of North American culture, against which he and his wife had to work.

Stories of self are vehicles for learning about self in time and in relation. A culture speaks through its members, who, via narratives of the self, reproduce it (Gergen & Gergen, 1988, p. 40), even if only to resist it. Such stories provide the "diachronic and relational" elements of the human science theories we prize (Gergen & Gergen, 1988, p. 53). Stories are most immediately renderings of the particular and concrete, but they are also, in form and substance, universal and generalizable. When a woman tells of her successful struggle with infertility, or a man tells of his struggle with cancer, we are listening not just to different stories, one about infertility and one about cancer, but also to two variations of one story: a progressive, victory story. We may abstract the common narrative features or rhetorical devices that are used to tell such victory stories. Because individuals use stories to describe and explain events and to justify themselves, we may see these stories as constituting their creators' descriptive, explanatory, and moral theories of how adversity—whether in the form of infertility or cancer—was, can be, or ought to be encountered and overcome. In this important sense, good stories are like good theories in making our world more understandable and predictable and in describing and even prescribing ways to act.

Truth/StoryTelling in Nursing

The stories we tell in our research reports and the stories we hear in research interviews comprise efforts to tell the truth. Stories are the "strategic" (Riessman, 1990) means by which human beings develop, sustain, and present definitions of self and reality. Until we acknowledge the truth in stories and realize that the goal of both theory and story construction is less to discover the Truth than to create it—to make sense, meaning, and order—we will continue to deceive ourselves.

Acknowledging the truth in stories and the storied nature of truth obliges us to preserve the integrity of the data we obtain in the typical qualitative research interview. Although "our analyses are always and inevitably disruptions" (Gergen, 1989, p. 66), a consciousness of the interview as narrative will make our analysis less disruptive of, and more faithful to, the whole story. Interview data are "never simply raw" but rather "situated and textual," not "naturally occurring" but rather "artifacts" of research (Silverman, 1989, pp. 218, 226). Accordingly, we cannot afford to forget the phenomenology of the interview situation itself in producing our phenomenologies, nor can we afford to forget the narrative ground of our grounded theories.

Furthermore, we cannot continue to fetishize techniques that will not further and are incompatible with our goals. We often talk of the plurality of truths, but we still often act as if there were only one Truth. We forget that there is no such thing as the "same" event; there is only an "event under a description" (Rosaldo, 1989, p. 136). We forget that the very act of telling the putatively same story is a retelling, resulting in the inappropriateness of making conventional efforts to ensure reliability and consensual validity. Indeed, as Silverman (1989) noted, efforts to "triangulate" interview data with other data are often "simple-minded" (p. 219) in ignoring not only the revisionist nature of storytelling but also the inherent differences between interview and other kinds of data.

Moreover, discrepancies between accounts, whether given by one person or different persons, ought not to be treated as if one of the accounts were wrong but rather ought to be considered as analytic directives to explain why and even whether they really are different. In this regard, consider Silverman's (1989) demonstration of how interview data not corroborated by other data may yet be seen as conveying truths. In his study of parents in a pediatric cardiology unit, Silverman observed that contrary to the parents' accounts of the physicians' consultation room being too crowded with other staff members to be conducive to their asking questions, parents actually asked more questions when more people were in the room. He did not treat this finding as evidence of the unreliability of these parents as informants or of the greater objectivity of the data he had collected showing the relationship between the actual numbers of questions parents asked and the actual numbers of staff present. Instead of dismissing the parents' accounts as uncorroborated explanations of their behavior, he recognized them as "moral tales" conveying the parents' struggle to be seen as responsible—as "situated appeals to the rationality and moral appropriateness of that behavior" (p. 219).

To bolster his demonstration, Silverman (1989) referred to the comparably dramatic and engaging "atrocity stories" told by patients in another study of physician-patient interactions. He argued that by means of these tales, patients were able to vent feelings, to redress perceived social inequalities, and to highlight their own rationality. Similarly, Blaxter (1983) argued that a medically "incorrect" statement concerning disease should be treated not as a mistake but as an invitation to examine preferred modes of explanation and the differences that exist between medical and lay models of disease.

Conclusion

Recognizing the truths, as opposed to the *lies/mistakes,* in tales means foregoing naive notions of stories as either true or false. It also enjoins us to develop our skills in the construction and analysis of narratives, just as we continue to refine them in the construction and analysis of theories. We must engage in some "strategic borrowing" (DeVault, 1990, p. 109) of approaches that we have to date associated exclusively with the biographer, historian, writer of fiction, and literary critic. The rules for and implications of such strategic borrowing in nursing research have yet to be fully developed, but the essentially biographical, historical, and storied nature of the interview data we collect demands such work. Importantly, we cannot hope to get either the whole story or the whole truth by attending only to the informational contents of interviews: by viewing lives-as-told as equal to lives-as-lived and lives-as-experienced (Bruner, 1984). Indeed, truths are found in the way people "compose" their lives (Bateson, 1989).

Note

1. A similar argument has been advanced concerning the conventional and deliberately dispassionate research report, which constrains the researcher to tell the truth in a certain way, thereby limiting what can be told. For example, the author is obliged to assume a third-person narrative stance, to separate method from findings, to separate findings from interpretation, and to make certain rhetorical appeals to the validity of process and product (Gusfield, 1976; Hunter, 1990).

References

Barley, N. (1988). *Not a hazardous sport.* New York: Holt.
Bateson, M. C. (1989). *Composing a life.* New York: Plume.
Blaxter, M. (1983). The causes of disease: Women talking. *Social Science and Medicine, 17,* 59-69.
Bloor, M. J. (1983). Notes on member validation. In R. M. Emerson (Ed.), *Contemporary field research: A collection of readings* (pp. 156-172). Boston: Little, Brown.
Bruner, E. M. (1984). Introduction: The opening up of anthropology. In S. Plattner & E. M. Bruner (Eds.), *Text, play, and story: The construction and reconstruction of self and society* (pp. 1-16). Washington, DC: American Ethnological Society.
Bruner, E. M. (1986). Ethnography as narrative. In V. W. Turner & E. M. Bruner (Eds.), *The anthropology of experience* (pp. 139-155). Urbana: University of Illinois Press.
Chandrasekhar, S. (1987). *Truth and beauty: Aesthetics and motivations in science.* Chicago: University of Chicago Press.
Deutscher, I. (1970). Looking backward: Case study on the progress of methodology in sociological research. In W. Filstead (Ed.), *Qualitative methodology: Firsthand involvement with the social world* (pp. 202-216). Chicago: Markham.
DeVault, M. L. (1990). Talking and listening from women's standpoint: Feminist strategies for interviewing and analysis. *Social Problems, 37,* 96-116.
Gergen, M. M. (1988). Narrative structures in social explanation. In C. Antaki (Ed.), *Analyzing everyday explanation: A casebook of methods* (pp. 94-112). London: Sage.
Gergen, M. M. (1989). Talking about menopause: A dialogic analysis. In L. E. Thomas (Ed.), *Research on adulthood and aging: The human sciences approach* (pp. 65-87). Albany: State University of New York Press.
Gergen, K. J., & Gergen, M. M. (1986). Narrative form and the construction of psychological science. In T. R. Sarbin (Ed.), *Narrative psychology: The storied nature of human conduct* (pp. 22-44). New York: Praeger.
Gergen, K. J., & Gergen, M. M. (1988). Narrative and the self as relationship. *Advances in Experimental Social Psychology, 21,* 17-56.
Goodman, N. (1978). *Ways of worldmaking.* Sussex, UK: Harvester.
Gusfield, J. (1976). The literary rhetoric of science: Comedy and pathos in drinking driver research. *American Sociological Review, 41,* 16-34.
Hospers, J. (1946). *Meaning and truth in the arts.* Chapel Hill: University of North Carolina Press.

Hunter, A. (1990). Introduction: Rhetoric in research, networks of knowledge. In A. Hunter (Ed.), *The rhetoric of social research: Understood and believed* (pp. 1-22). New Brunswick, NJ: Rutgers University Press.

Kirk, J., & Miller, M. L. (1986). *Reliability and validity in qualitative research.* Beverly Hills, CA: Sage.

Krieger, S. (1991). *Social science and the self: Personal essays on an art form.* New Brunswick, NJ: Rutgers University Press.

Mishler, E. G. (1990). Validation in inquiry-guided research: The role of exemplars in narrative studies. *Harvard Educational Review, 60,* 415-442.

Morgan, G. (1983). Exploring choice: Reframing the process of evaluation. In G. Morgan (Ed.), *Beyond method: Strategies for social research* (pp. 392-404). Beverly Hills, CA: Sage.

Nisbet, R. (1976). *Sociology as an art form.* New York: Oxford University Press.

Personal Narratives Group. (1989). Truths. In Personal Narratives Group (Ed.), *Interpreting women's lives: Feminist theory and personal narratives* (pp. 261-264). Bloomington: Indiana University Press.

Richardson, L. (1990a). Narrative and sociology. *Journal of Contemporary Ethnography, 19,* 116-135.

Richardson, L. (1990b). *Writing strategies: Reaching diverse audiences.* Newbury Park, CA: Sage.

Riessman, C. K. (1987). When gender is not enough: Women interviewing women. *Gender and Society, 1,* 172-207.

Riessman, C. K. (1990). Strategic uses of narrative in the presentation of self and illness: A research note. *Social Science and Medicine, 30,* 1195-1200.

Robinson, J. A., & Hawpe, L. (1986). Narrative thinking as a heuristic process. In T. R. Sarbin (Ed.), *Narrative psychology: The storied nature of human conduct* (pp. 111-125). New York: Praeger.

Rosaldo, R. (1989). *Culture and truth: The remaking of social analysis.* Boston: Beacon.

Rosenwald, G. C. (1988). A theory of multiple-case research. In D. P. McAdams & R. L. Ochberg (Eds.), *Psychobiography and life narratives* (pp. 239-264). Durham, NC: Duke University Press.

Sandelowski, M. (1991). Telling stories: Narrative approaches in qualitative research. *Image, 23,* 161-166.

Sandelowski, M., Holditch-Davis, D., & Harris, B. G. (1990). Living the life: Explanations of infertility. *Sociology of Health and Illness, 12,* 195-215.

Silverman, D. (1989). Six rules of qualitative research: A post-romantic argument. *Symbolic Interaction, 12,* 215-230.

Spence, D. P. (1982). *Narrative truth and historical truth: Meaning and interpretation in psychoanalysis.* New York: Norton.

Tirrell, L. (1990). Storytelling and moral agency. *Journal of Aesthetics and Art Criticism, 48,* 115-126.

Walker, L. O., & Avant, K. C. (1988). *Strategies for theory construction in nursing* (2nd ed.). Norwalk, CT: Appleton & Lange.

Watson, L. C. (1976). Understanding a life history as a subjective document. *Ethos, 4,* 95-131.

Watson, L. C. (1989). The question of "individuality" in life history interpretation. *Ethos, 17,* 308-325.

CHAPTER 10

Poeticizing as Truth
in Nursing Inquiry

JEAN WATSON

We are well aware that poetry has a place in our life—the life of the mind, imagination, and evocation. We may eventually consider poetry to be a way of, a form of, knowing. But then what is its relation to that most fundamental pursuit—the search for Truth and Truth itself? What is Truth? And what does poetry have to do with Truth? In seeking answers to such questions, it is important to keep in mind Parker's (1987) statement that we must be careful in our development of

AUTHOR'S NOTE: This chapter, originally presented on May 5, 1993, at the "Philosophy in the Nurse's World" conference, is adapted, with permission of the National League for Nursing Press, from "Poeticizing as Truth Through Language," by Jean Watson, in *Art and Aesthetics in Nursing* (F. L. Chinn & J. Watson, Eds.). Copyright © 1994 by National League for Nursing Press.

knowledge and Truth because we shape souls by the nature of our knowledge: We can form or deform human souls.

The Pursuit of Truth

The pursuit of Truth (with a capital "T") is, beyond question, in the world of science. Surely we must not interfere with that pursuit, even if we enjoy our own experience with poetry. So, then, is poetry better placed outside the world of Truth and science? I suppose the ontology of knowing that characterizes Western world science and could be labeled as "separatist" would have us take that position. Indeed, in this conventional ontology, it is held that "the truth of any proposition (its factual quality) can be determined by testing it empirically in the natural world. Any proposition that has withstood such a test is True; such Truth is absolute" (Guba & Lincoln, 1989, p. 104). Within this perspective, it is thought that Truth follows appropriate inquiry or methodology—namely, the conducting of experiments in a value-free context—resulting in what Guba and Lincoln (1989) suggested is the ritual of method. With regard to the problem of the primacy of method, Nietzsche (cited in Gadamer, 1988) stated, "It is not the victory of science that distinguishes this century, but the victory of scientific method over science" (p. xii).

However, as participants in a search for Truth, we do not, and cannot, stand outside the world of method of Truth making. Even phenomenology, as a liberating approach for human science, was originally conceived within the natural science paradigm and thus reflects a tendency toward dominance of method (Gadamer, 1988). Indeed, in his book entitled *Truth and Method,* Gadamer (1960/1991) sought to show the drawbacks of methodology's rule within the human sciences, turning to the arts and poetry as a means of gaining access to an irresistible Truth overlooked in the dogmatic application of method. Gadamer (1960/1991) reminded us that Truth is not necessarily discovered *without,* but by interpretation and meaning. He explained that the contemporary ontological shift that has occurred with hermeneutics is guided by language—language as experience of the world and as horizon of a hermeneutic ontology.

Because we are humans, our truths are co-created through a process involving both values and meaning making, using language. When our values become human values of caring for self, others, and all living things, including the planet Earth, and when the meaning making of Truth involves humans and the co-creation of meaning through language, then a scenario becomes possible within which we can consider poeticizing as Truth.

The different scenario of the co-creation of Truth through language, experience, and meaning making becomes possible precisely because we as humans have a choice among ways of knowing, being, and doing Truth. However, we as humans do not have the option not to seek Truth, of "not knowing, because it is the nature of beings like us with subjectivity to use language to formulate meanings" (Gadow, 1990, p. 2), to come to some Truth within our world and ourselves. In this regard, Merleau Ponty (1962) reminded us that we are given to ourselves as something to be understood. And, as Heidegger (1971) put it, our being hears the call of language that speaks of the being of all things that respond to a mortal language that speaks of what it hears. Thus, because knowing through language and Truth seeking are part of our being, we cannot help being part of this process.

Nonetheless, we can decide whether the Truth we seek shall be a means of concealment, a means of refusing or disengaging from life, accomplishing, for us, our distance from the world (Gadow, 1990). If we opt for distance and nonlife, for what Heidegger (1971) called *concealment* (i.e., an object-stance relationship with the world), then we have also opted for the model of Truth and knowing that science for centuries has chosen (Gadow, 1990). Such a model of Truth making requires a one-to-one correspondence theory of Truth (i.e., a direct, linear relationship between facts and the physical universe) and the use of a language of concealment. If we adopt the object-stance model, we give up choice of values; subjective, imaginative, and evocative meanings; and, as Hofstadter (1971) stated, our "authentic relationship as mortal to other mortals, to earth and sky, to the divinities present or absent, to things and plants and animals" (p. x). But perhaps equally important is the effect of our choice on the Beauty-Truth correspondence associated with the *aletheia* theory of Truth.

Unconcealedness and Truth

For Heidegger (1971), as for me, the nature of Truth is found in the Greek word *aletheia,* meaning, for Heidegger, "the unconcealment of beings" (pp. 50-51). Unconcealedness occurs in the open place in the midst of beings, the clearing that is created. However, the clearing is never set. Rather, the clearing happens only as a double concealment; it is never a merely existent state, but a happening. From this, we begin to see that unconcealedness, meaning "Truth" for Heidegger, is not an attribute of factual things, in the sense of beings. We begin to see, too, that "Truth in its nature, is un-truth" (Heidegger, 1971, p. 54). However, that does not mean that Truth is falsehood, nor does it mean that Truth is never itself; rather, it means that Truth, viewed dialectically, is always also its opposite.

With these circular ambiguities, perhaps we may ask, as does Heidegger (1971), "How does Truth happen?" Heidegger stated that it happens when that which is as a whole is brought into unconcealedness and "held" therein—with the word *held (huten)* originally meaning "kept, taken care of." In the way that Truth happens in, say, Van Gogh's painting of the shoes, "this does not mean everything is correctly portrayed, but rather that in the revelation of the being of the shoes, that which is as a whole—world and earth in their counterplay—attains to unconcealedness" (Heidegger, 1971, p. 56).

If we choose to opt for concealment, as has science, we eliminate the Beauty-Truth correspondence associated with the *aletheia* theory of Truth, which embraces the spirit of Truth as well as the direct, open, and unfolding relationship between Beauty and Truth. This relationship is depicted by John Keats (1819/1983) in his *Ode on a Grecian Urn:*

> *"Beauty is truth, truth beauty"—that is all*
> *Ye know on earth, and all ye need to know.*
> *(p. 644)*

If we can identify with Keats through poetry as a form of Truth and Beauty, we can rejoin the world as inhabitants, open to our being, which includes human language and aesthetics. We can sense Arthur

Koestler's (1968) *Ghost in the Machine* at the same time we cope with Marx's (1964) *Machine in the Garden*. If we can cross over into the world of authentic being and hold ourselves open to its being, then we can experience and reside in both outer and inner self-evident Truth, not as aliens, separate from and separated from our own Truth, but as authentic residents.

The difference between concealedness and unconcealedness is the difference between the following passage from Denise Levertov's (1967/1983) *The Closed World:*

> *"If the Perceptive Organs close, their Objects seem to close also."*
> —*Blake: Jerusalem*
> *The house-snake dwells here still*
> *under the threshold*
> *but for months I have not seen it*
> *nor its young, the inheritors.*
> *Light and the wind enact*
> *passion and resurrection*
> *day in, day out*
> *but the blinds are down over my windows,*
> *my doors are shut.*
>
> (pp. 1248-1249)[1]

and this passage from Ammons's (1971/1983) *Poetics:*

> *I look for the way*
> *things will turn*
> *out spiraling from a center,*
> *the shape*
> *things will take to come forth in*
> *so that the birch tree white*
> *touched black at branches*
> *will stand out*
> *wind-glittering*
> *totally its apparent self.*
> *I look for the forms*
> *things want to come as*
> *from what black wells of possibility,*
> *how a thing will*
> *unfold;*

. . .
not so much looking for the shape
as being available
to any shape that may be
summoning itself
through me
from the self not mine but ours.
                    (pp. 1258-1259)[2]

These two works help us to see the difference between the con-
cealed/closed model of Truth and the poetic/unconcealed model of
Truth. We see, too, the unconcealedness of poetry as Truth about
which Heidegger (1971) wrote so extensively.

Poetic Truth

In Heidegger's view (1971), the speech of genuine thinking is by
nature *poetic*. It need not take the shape of verse because the opposite
of poetry is not prose; pure prose is as poetic as any poetry. As
Heidegger (1971) stated, "The voice of thought must be poetic
because poetry is the saying of Truth, the saying of the unconcealedness of beings. . . . Poetry that thinks is in truth the topology of being.
This topology tells Being the whereabouts of its actual presence"
(p. 12).

According to Gadamer (1988), it is the art of language that determines not only the success or failure of poetry but also its claim to
Truth. The old Platonic objection to the trustworthiness of poetry and
poets—"Poets often lie"—is opposite to the belief in the truthfulness
of art generally; this claim is not easily silenced (p. 106). However,
though indeed it has been said that poets often lie to get at Truth, their
language is haunting and will not be silenced because poetry is the
language of people.

Within the *aletheia* view of Truth, "the task of poetry is to instruct
as well as to please" (Hofstadter, quoted in Heidegger, 1971, p. x).
Thus poetry is a valid endeavor in both classical aesthetics and
contemporary science—at least in a human science that elicits a
reflective form of Truth, co-constituted in a mortal language that

speaks of what it hears and experiences (Hofstadter, cited in Heidegger, 1971, p. x).

Just as there is Truth in art, so, too, there is Truth in poetry. The poem that Heidegger describes as portraying a "Roman fountain," or the poem that says, "so much depends / upon / a red wheel / barrow / glazed with rain / water / beside the white / chickens" (Williams, 1923/1983, p. 945),[2] does not

> just make manifest . . . anything at all; rather, [it] make[s] unconcealedness as such happen in regard to what is as a whole. The more simply and authentically the [items] are engrossed in their nature, the more directly and engagingly do all beings attain to a greater degree of being along with them. That is how self-concealing being is illuminated. Light of this kind joins its shining to and into the work. This shining, joined in the work, is the beautiful. *Beauty is one way in which truth occurs as unconcealedness.* (Heidegger, 1971, p. 56)

In William Carlos Williams's (1923/1983) poem "Red Wheel Barrow," we see Heidegger's position (1971) that the nature of Truth is the unconcealedness of beings; that is the nature of being (p. xxi).

When we invert the closed world of Truth in which we conceal and are cut off from our world, and when we consider poeticizing as Truth, we recover a world of Truth in which we have a place and in which things, in a world that is assumed to be inexhaustible and not closed or limited, are opened up to us, unfolded to us (Gadow, 1990, p. 14). But "there is no getting to the end of it because we know it now through language of poetry from within, not from outside" (Gadow, 1990, p. 14).

In this world that we can know from the inside through language and poetry, there can be no falseness because there is no external standard against which language and poetry can be measured and to which they must correspond. Yet this world is far from arbitrary. It represents a unique kind of risk, for it can fail to live up to itself. In poetry, Truth may fail to happen not because it fails to correspond to "facts," but because its work proves to be "empty." According to Gadamer (1988), poetry is "empty" when, instead of sounding right, it merely sounds like other poetry or like the rhetoric of everyday life; when the work fulfills itself and becomes language, we must take it at its word (p. 139). Poetry is not fulfilled by anything beyond itself—that is, by any confirmation we might seek through verification of facts or through further experience. Poetry fulfills itself (Gadamer, 1988, p. 111). "Poetically man Dwells" (Heidegger, 1971, p. xxi).

At the same time that poetry fulfills itself, and we dwell in it as our being, poetic language and the poetic word evoke the idea of something beyond, for example, the literal "fountain" or "wheel barrow." We do not look in the direction of any particular fountain or wheelbarrow; rather, each of us constructs an image of a fountain or wheelbarrow in a way that it stands there for each of us as "the Roman fountain" or "the red wheel barrow." As such, we construct the world of the poem from within the poem itself, provoking an immediate refusal to seek verification of what is said, heard, or read. According to Gadamer (1988), one of the reasons for this refusal is that a genuine poem allows us to experience "nearness" in such a way that this nearness is held in and through the linguistic form of the poem. In other words, although fundamental human experiences always change and are constantly subject to change, "the poem does not fade, for the poetic word brings the transience of time to a standstill. . . . It stands written, where its own presence is in play. This standing of the work is related to the fundamental situation that Hegel described as feeling at home in the world" (Gadamer, 1988, p. 114). As Gadamer (1988) explained, the poem not only helps us in "making ourselves at home" but also stands over against this, holding the world up to us like a mirror.

> But what appears in this mirror is not the world, nor this or that thing in the world, but rather, this nearness or familiarity itself in which we stand for a while. . . . This is but a description of the fact that language gives all of us our access to a world in which certain special forms of human experience arise; . . . the poetic word that by being there bears witness to our own being. (p. 115)

In the next part of this chapter, I discuss poetry as method at the uniquely human level and at the disciplinary level. In both instances, the object-stance paradigm is inverted, and Truth is pursued from the inside out—in terms of the unconcealed model rather than the closed/concealed model of traditional systems. As a result, not only are new clearings opened but there is evidence of poeticizing itself as a form of Truth. This Truth through poeticizing embraces knowing from the inside out and elicits a form of Truth as Beauty that stands for itself. It is such Truth that nursing seeks through its engaged inquiry into subjective and intersubjective human caring and healing experiences.

Poetry as Method

As part of the postmodern constructivist mood to ground human science as method, science and even some forms of feminist scholarship, poetry, story, and narrative have all been used as ways to decenter the unreflexive self to create a position for experiencing the self as an engaged knower/constructor. As such, poetry has been revealed to be a way to (re)write the self as well as to unite people's (inter)subjective experiences with one's own interpretations.

POSTMODERN TURN

One contemporary approach to considering poetry as a form of Truth is to take, as its subject matter, the lived experience of the researcher rather than external data per se. Considering the life world of the researcher is part of an epistemic shift within and across disciplines that joins the growing genre of research that is framed as interpretive biography (Denzin, 1989), ethnographic fiction (Richardson, 1992), radical hermeneutics (Caputo, 1987), radical empiricism (Jackson, 1989), transcendental phenomenology (Levin, 1983; Watson, 1985, 1995), interpretive hermeneutics (Gadamer, 1988; Habermas, 1983), story as method, and so on. This interpretative turn is one of the consequences of the disenchantment with the "modern structuralist era" of science and scientism, which we are now leaving behind as we enter the postmodern era. But more important, this contemporary postmodern turn is a search for ontological and epistemological authenticity as a form of Truth, with respect to both the phenomenon of interest and its human expression (Guba & Lincoln, 1989; Lincoln & Guba, 1985).

Ontological authenticity is specifically at issue in the human-to-human transpersonal and contextual field, within which nursing research, as praxis, finds itself with respect to the conditions and experiences of being human. For example, while the nurse researcher, functioning within the qualitative research paradigms—phenomenology, ethnoscience, hermeneutics, and so on—attempts to capture the descriptive meaning of the subjective lived experiences of patients, empirical traditional science looms over him or her, keeping the focus external (even though it is subjective). There remains a focusing on the "other out there," and not much attention is paid to the transaction per se. If the transaction is considered, it is as secondary to the phenomenon of interest and only as a means of informing the researcher about the other's experience.

In contrast, within a postmodern frame, and in considering poeticizing as Truth, it is acknowledged that it is never possible to know another person's experience. Even though we may intuit it or vicariously identify with it, it remains uniquely *other*. However, it is thought that perhaps the closest we can come to knowing the other's experience is to become better acquainted with how the other's experience is reflected onto us—as researcher, as clinician, and so on. Thus we set up a whole new dynamic of understanding human experience through direct access to how the researcher is experiencing the human condition reflected onto him or her.

By inverting the paradigm for understanding human experiences—that is, by understanding from the inside out—we come full circle, from modern, detached, sterile language to postmodern connections, interpretations, and aesthetics, in seeing how it is possible to take, as nursing's subject matter, the lived experience of the nurse and authentically and even poetically to express it as such. With this ontological and epistemic turn, nursing research(ers) can be conceptually consistent with the postmodern shift being made by researchers in many other disciplines. Further, this postmodern turn allows nursing to be ontologically and epistemologically authentic with respect to both its history and its tradition as well as with its most contemporary subject matter of human caring, healing, and health experiences. In so doing, another consideration arises related to treatment of the subjective human experience data of the researcher. This is perhaps where the postmodern question related to poeticizing and Truth comes most dramatically into play.

Transcendentally, authentic languaging—the conscious, selective use of language to elicit feeling and evoke an inner kind of knowing— is involved in the potential for growth implied in our lived and felt transaction within the research experience as well as in our reflection upon experience. This experiential difference is not so much a question of different contexts of meaning as it is a question of ways of relating to the experiential process. For example, an aboriginal does not own land, but the land owns him. The two kinds of relationship are entirely different. How the phenomenon experienced is reflected onto the nurse and then expressed is what is being questioned. Can something be poetic and still be true?

POETICIZING

Once one seeks ontological and epistemological authenticity with regard to the human experience in question, one has to consider authentic languaging to capture the experience. Heidegger (1971) urged that we actually undergo an experience with language and let experiences speak for themselves. In the process, we should let our- selves be transformed by our participation. For Heidegger (1971), the result is poeticizing. If the researcher engages in and is reflective of the depth of the human experience and is true to the moving human experience, he or she almost naturally poeticizes, and the result cannot be other than poetic. Levin (1983) noted that in phenomenological discourse, "The deepest transcendental truth of an existentially authentic languaging of experience will be articulated naturally with the sensuous resonance, the emotional spaciousness, and the elemental openness of the poetic word" (pp. 228, 229).

With respect to the Truth of poeticizing around human experiences, in acknowledging the authenticity and transcendental nature of both the experience and our expression of it, it is necessary also to acknow- ledge that the way in which experience is expressed is at least as important as the content, the facts, and the pure description of the experience. In other words, how can cold, unfeeling, and totally detached dogmatic words and tone possibly convey the Truth or deep

meaning of a human phenomenon associated with human and transpersonal caring—the sorrow, great beauty, passion, and joy found
there (Watson, 1985, pp. 91-93)? We cannot convey complexity or the
need for compassion or cultivate feeling and sensibility in words that
are bereft of warmth, kindness, and good feeling. Within the postmodern paradigm, there exists poetic ambiguity of human life itself.
But this ambiguity is what brings Truth of an experience into being—
poeticizing as a form of Truth telling that is authentic to the poetic
ambiguity. To quote Levin (1983),

> If there be any truth, then [in the method], it must be that the transcen-
> dental is not just a method for understanding the facticity of experience;
> but that it is also a way of enjoying, or appreciating the intrinsically
> creative and open nature of experiences, because appreciation of this
> nature is a necessary condition for true and authentic existential knowl-
> edge. (p. 221)

Conclusion

If we are to consider the deep level of human experiences and
transactions, we can adopt the *aletheia* theory of Truth. Human
science and art of nursing and human caring and healing, which are
deeply transpersonal, can incorporate feeling and authentic experiential language. The expression of the healing experience can only be
poetic because it possesses its own Truth by bringing the experience
into being. In turn, it reminds us that as nurses, educators, practitioners, or researchers, we are first of all human beings, capable both of
being fully embodied in a caring moment and of transcending the
moment, expressing it with the depth and beauty it calls forth from
us and in us.

If we indeed consider poeticizing as Truth, then we acknowledge
that we are participants in a postmodern era that is engaged in a search
for new forms of authentic Truth searching and Truth making—an era
that seeks connections, meanings, and subjective and aesthetic expressions, all of which contribute to the shaping of multiple truths about
human phenomena and human meanings related to caring, healing,
and health experiences and relations. These new, yet old, forms of

Truth searching include a search for scientific Truth—ontological, epistemological, and methodological authenticity; more adherence to the *aletheia* theory of Truth, the Truth of unfoldment; an expansion and fusing of horizons of meaning; and a search for fit between phenomena and forms of expression.

Watson (1995) stated that as we make the postmodern turn, which incidentally reconnects us with art and science as well as the ancient traditions of science that accommodated matter and metaphysics, we move from

- the analytic to the poetic
- the descriptive to the interpretative
- phenomena per se to experience, story, being, and relation
- the ontic/the entities/elements to the thing itself/the ontological
- structure to process
- data and facts to text-narrative and connections
- numbers to words, language, text, and meaning
- object-object or object-subject to intersubjectivity and subjectivity as Truth telling

As we become part of the postmodern turn, we can do no other than enter the dance of poeticizing as we construct Truth. We construct this new-found subjectivist Truth by way of expanding our horizons of meaning and insights. We discover this Truth by fully actualizing our past and our new-found future that is embedded in humanity, human meanings, language, and experience. And, finally, we enter into this poetic Truth as a form of poetic justice as we reconnect with whom and what we have become as humans—co-creators of ourselves and our discipline, just as we are co-creators of science and art. As we make this final turn, we now know that we own a new Truth, a Truth not only that we have created but in which we can dwell.

Notes

1. William Carlos Williams: *Collected Poems: 1909-1939, Volume I.* Copyright © 1938 by New Directions Publishing Corp. Reprinted by permission of New Directions Publishing Corporation and Laurence Pollinger Limited.

2. Reprinted from *Collected Poems 1951-1971* by A. R. Ammons, with the permission of W. W. Norton & Company, Inc. Copyright © 1971 by A. R. Ammons.
3. Denise Levertov: *Relearning the Alphabet.* Copyright © 1966 by Denise Levertov. Reprinted by permission of New Directions Publishing Corp.

References

Ammons, A. R. (1983). *Poetics.* In A. W. Allison, H. Barrows, C. Blake, A. Carr, A. Eastman, & H. M. English (Eds.), *Norton Anthology of Poetry* (pp. 1258-1259). New York: Norton. (Original work published 1971)

Caputo, J. D. (1987). *Radical hermeneutics.* Indianapolis: Indiana University Press.

Denzin, N. K. (1989). *Interpretive biography.* Newbury Park, CA: Sage.

Gadamer, H. G. (1988). *The relevance of the beautiful and other essays* (R. Bernasconi, Ed.). New York: Cambridge University Press.

Gadamer, H. G. (1991). *Truth and method* (2nd ed.). New York: Crossroad. (Original work published 1960)

Gadow, S. (1990). *Beyond dualism: The dialectic of caring and knowing.* Paper presented at the Conference "Caring: A Call to Consciousness," Houston, TX.

Guba, E., & Lincoln, Y. (1989). *Fourth generation evaluation.* Newbury Park, CA: Sage.

Habermas, J. (1983). *Knowledge and human interests* (J. J. Shapiro, Trans.). Boston: Beacon.

Heidegger, M. (1971). *Poetry, language, thought* (A. Hofstadter, Trans.). New York: Harper & Row.

Hofstadter, A. (1971). Introduction. In M. Heidegger, *Poetry, language, thought* (A. Hofstadter, Trans., p. x). New York: Harper & Row.

Jackson, M. (1989). *Paths toward a clearing: Radical empiricism and ethnographic inquiry.* Indianapolis: University of Indiana Press.

Keats, J. (1983). *Ode on a Grecian urn.* In A. W. Allison, H. Barrows, C. Blake, A. Carr, A. Eastman, & H. M. English (Eds.), *Norton anthology of poetry* (p. 664). New York: Norton. (Original work published 1819)

Koestler, A. (1968). *Ghost in the machine.* New York: Macmillan.

Levertov, D. (1983). *The closed world.* In A. W. Allison, H. Barrows, C. Blake, A. Carr, A. Eastman, & H. M. English (Eds.), *Norton anthology of poetry* (pp. 1248-1249). New York: Norton. (Original work published 1967)

Levin, D. (1983). The poetic function in phenomenological discourse. In W. L. McBride & C. O. Schrag (Eds.), *Phenomenology in a pluralistic context* (pp. 216-234). Albany: State University of New York Press.

Lincoln, Y. S., & Guba, E. C. (1985). *Naturalistic inquiry.* Beverly Hills, CA: Sage.

Marx, L. (1964). *Machine in the garden: Technology and the pastoral ideal in America.* New York: Oxford University Press.

Merleau Ponty, M. (1962). *Phenomenology of perception.* London: Routledge & Kegan Paul.

Parker, P. (1987). Community, conflict, and ways of knowing. *Magazine of Higher Education, 19,* 20-25.

Richardson, L. (1992). The consequences of poetic representation: Writing the other, rewriting the self. In C. Ellis & G. Flaherty [Eds.), *Investigating subjectivity: Research on lived experience* (pp. 125-141). Newbury Park, CA: Sage.

Watson, J. (1985). *Nursing: Human science and human care.* New York: National League for Nursing.

Watson, J. (1995). Postmodernism and knowledge development in nursing. *Nursing Science Quarterly, 8*(2), 60-64.

Williams, W. C. (1983). *Red wheel barrow.* In A. W. Allison, H. Barrows, C. Blake, A. Carr, A. Eastman, & H. M. English (Eds.), *Norton anthology of poetry* (p. 945). New York: Norton. (Original work published 1923)

CHAPTER 11

Problems Inherent in the Epistemology and Methodologies of Feminist Research

DONNA M. ROMYN

The women's movement and an increasing awareness of women's health issues have led to the emergence of feminist research within the nursing discipline. MacPherson (1983) noted that this development represents a paradigm shift in nursing science. She claimed that the scientific paradigm used previously by nurse researchers did not allow for the exploration of women's experiences, including phenomena such as wife battering during pregnancy or the homicide of women. Nor did it allow for feminist critique.

Underlying this paradigm shift is an assumption that feminist research is more than the study of women (Chinn, 1981, 1989; McBride, 1984). Webb (1993) defined feminist research as being "research *on*

140

women, *by* women, *for* women" (p. 422). Feminist research focuses on questions related to understanding the conditions of women's lives and delineating the causes and consequences of women's oppression. Feminist theory offers descriptions of women's oppression and prescriptions for eliminating it (MacPherson, 1983). The essence of feminist research and theory lies in their goals: increasing awareness, sensitization, and advocacy for change in social, political, and health policies that affect women (Parker & McFarlane, 1991).

Increasingly, research based on feminist theory is being published in the nursing literature. However, to date, there has been little critical examination of the epistemological assumptions and related feminist methodologies underlying the research or of their implications for the development of nursing knowledge and nursing practice. This chapter concerns the adequacy of the underpinnings of feminist research. What is at issue here is not whether oppression of women exists but rather whether feminist research, as currently grounded, can generate the nursing knowledge required to intervene in relation to that oppression. I will argue that problems inherent in the epistemological and methodological underpinnings of feminist research (as described in the nursing literature) are such that if they are left unresolved, the possibility of attaining the knowledge required to eliminate women's oppression is preempted.

My argument is based on the assumption that nursing is a practice discipline and that nursing knowledge is developed with a view toward improving nursing practice. Whereas the aim of an academic discipline is to know and its theories are descriptive in nature, a practice discipline is directed toward practical aims and thus generates prescriptive as well as descriptive theories (Donaldson & Crowley, 1978/1992, p. 208). Further, it is assumed that research and practice have different functions in the nursing discipline. The function of research is to attain theories to inform practice, whereas practice uses the theories generated by research to guide its activities in the particular case. In arguing, I will make explicit the principal epistemological assumptions and related methodologies underlying feminist research and will identify the problems inherent in them for the development of nursing knowledge. To begin, key terms including *epistemology, methodology,* and *methods* are defined, and the role of each in the development of knowledge is identified.

Epistemology, Methodology, and Method

Harding (1987) noted that questions and controversies in feminist inquiry stem from confusion in the meanings of the terms *method, methodology,* and *epistemology.* For example, questions such as "Can quantitative research be feminist in orientation?" "Are only qualitative research approaches appropriate for the investigation of feminist phenomena?" and "Is there a method of inquiry that is distinctly feminist?" are indicative of one of the major controversies: the relationship between feminist ideology and research methods (Campbell & Bunting, 1991).

Epistemology, the theory of knowledge, determines the assumptions underlying a particular methodology. Questions of an epistemological nature concern what can be known and who can be a knower and the criteria by which beliefs are judged and considered to be knowledge. Methodology is simply a theory of how research should proceed (Harding, 1987). The manner in which techniques for gathering information are used is an issue of methodology, not of method. Thus the assertion, by feminists, that scientists have chosen to study phenomena from an essentially male perspective is a critique of epistemology and methodology rather than of method (Campbell & Bunting, 1991). Harding (1987) defined *method* as a technique for gathering information and noted that it is not method(s) but rather the unique purpose of the inquiry and the relationships established between the researcher and the informant that make feminist research distinctive. She argued that although methods can be subsumed under observation, dialogue with informants, or examination of records, they are not bound to a particular philosophical stance. She correctly stated that methods can be used from the perspective of any worldview and are not driven by the assumptions underlying a particular methodology. That is, they are not driven by the epistemology underlying a particular methodology.

Epistemology of Feminist Research

Feminist research is based upon an epistemological stance that holds that women's experiences are a legitimate source of knowledge and that women can be knowers (Campbell & Bunting, 1991). Whereas some nurse scholars hold that female gender is neither necessary nor sufficient for the conduct of feminist research (Campbell & Bunting, 1991; Webb, 1993), others argue that the principal investigator must be a woman (Duffy, 1985; Kremer, 1990; Parker & McFarlane, 1991). The latter argument implies that the attainment of knowledge is gender specific and that men cannot understand the experiences of women as described by women (and, conversely, that women cannot understand the experiences of men as described by men). If this perspective were held to be correct, men, including male nurses, would be precluded by virtue of gender from the development and utilization of feminist knowledge. Women, including female nurses, would assume sole responsibility not only for describing their own oppression but also for developing strategies to eliminate that oppression. A central question regarding this perspective is whether individuals, irrespective of gender, can develop sensitivity to feminist perspectives. Hall and Stevens (1991) stated that a "feminist conception of research for women does not provide a perspective that is immediately available to all women and only to women. Instead, it offers a way of conceptualizing reality that reflects women's interests and values and draws on women's own interpretations of their experiences" (p. 17).

Knowledge, in feminist research, is considered to be contextual and phenomena centered, and an intimate link is assumed to exist between the knower and what is to be known (Doering, 1992). Subjective data are considered to be valid, and knowledge is held to be relational, that is, mutually constructed between persons (Campbell & Bunting, 1991). In defining knowledge as relational, it is presupposed that there is no reality that exists independent of the mind and that knowledge is a matter of context and perspective rather than of objective truth (Schultz & Meleis, 1988, p. 220). Further, what is experienced is thought to be true, and hence individual descriptions of experiences are accepted as knowledge. In addition, the potential for multiple realities is assumed (Dzurec, 1989; Hall & Stevens, 1991). If this view were held to be correct, the knowledge generated by feminist nursing research would consist only of individual accounts of women's experiences. All accounts, whether contrary or not, would be held as true because there would be no objective reality against which the truth or falsity of a particular account could be measured. Further, differences of opinion related to the causes and consequences of women's oppression could not be resolved.

Viewing knowledge as contextual and relational has important implications for nursing practice. The practice of nursing would not have generalizable knowledge, in the form of descriptive and prescriptive theories, to guide it. More particularly, in the case of feminist theory, generalizable practical scientific knowledge of means to achieve the stated goals of empowering women and eliminating oppression would not exist. Bereft of the power of generalizability, nursing practitioners could not use the findings of research conducted with patients or clients other than their own (Schumacher & Gortner, 1992), and intervention in each practice situation would be the result of trial and error.

Although knowledge, in terms of women's experiences, is held to be contextual and relational in feminist research, certain moral values, such as those related to freedom from oppression and justice in the treatment of women, are not. Moral relativism was rejected by Thompson (1991), and MacPherson (1983) stated that what is good, true, and right for women is of concern to feminist researchers. A question that must be asked is whether it is possible to hold the position that knowledge is contextual and relational while simultaneously arguing that universal values exist related, for example, to justice in the treatment of women. It would seem that these two positions are contrary and that it would not be possible to hold both simultaneously. The existence of values that are applicable to all women presupposes the existence of a nature common to all women (an aspect of reality that is independent of the mind), a position that would be denied by many feminist theorists. This issue requires debate, given its implications for the development of a sound epistemological framework for feminist research and practice and for the development of research methodologies that are consistent with that epistemology.

Methodologies of Feminist Research

Methodologies that are described in the nursing literature as being based upon a feminist epistemology include feminist participatory research (Thompson, 1991), new paradigm research (Connors, 1988; MacPherson, 1983; Webb, 1984), and reflexivity (Anderson, 1991; Hall & Stevens, 1991; Harding, 1987). In each, women's experiences are afforded primacy, and the goal is taken to be understanding rather than control and affecting liberating change rather than maintaining the status quo. The research process is characterized by negotiation, reciprocity, and empowerment of both the researcher and the research participant (Connors, 1988). Empowerment of researcher and participant occurs through engagement in the research process (Anderson, 1991; Connors, 1988; Hall & Stevens, 1991; Thompson, 1991). The relationship between the researcher and the participant is nonhierarchical, nonauthoritarian, and nonmanipulative (Connors, 1988). Ownership and power with respect to the process and the product of the research are shared. Research participants engage in dialogue with the researcher to determine the research question(s) and process, to interpret the data, and to determine the content and process for the dissemination of findings to lay and professional groups (Connors, 1988; MacPherson, 1983; Parker & McFarlane, 1991; Seibold, Richards, & Simon, 1994; Thompson, 1991).

Feminist methodologies often include a research process whereby the values of the researcher are made explicit and become part of the research data (Campbell & Bunting, 1991; Parker & McFarlane, 1991). In the process, the researcher can determine the effects these values may have on the research process (Hall & Stevens, 1991) and can come to a better understanding of (her)self and the research participant(s) (Connors, 1988). The researcher becomes an active participant in the research and, in the process of conducting the research, often provides information to the participants as a means of empowerment. The experiences of both researcher and participant are changed as a result of participating in the research process, and that change becomes part of the data to be analyzed. This process is sometimes termed "research as praxis" (Chinn, 1989; Connors, 1988;

Thompson, 1991). Such descriptions of research as praxis raise two particularly important questions that have not been adequately addressed in the feminist nursing literature.

The first question is concerned with the relationship between research and practice. If the intent of research is to inform practice, how can research inform practice if research becomes practice, and practice, research? Can practice inform itself? Are not the objectives of research and practice different? Describing research as praxis creates undue blurring between the discipline and the practice of nursing (Batey, 1991). With this blurring, would the knowledge generated by the discipline of nursing not be the same as that generated in practice (i.e., knowledge of the particular)? And, in the case of feminist nursing research, would nursing practitioners not, once again, be left without the generalizable knowledge required to guide practice in working with women who are oppressed?

Second, if there is no reality that exists independent of the mind and no knowledge that is generalizable, on what basis does the researcher determine that certain groups of women (and not others) are oppressed and require intervention? Further, if knowledge is relational and the research participant—say, a battered wife—participates in interpretation of the data and insists that she is not oppressed, what implications does this have for research as praxis? Does the research, as praxis, terminate? If not, then would the researcher not have to apply general knowledge of oppression in this particular case to proceed? It is unclear how such apparent contradictions are resolved when action on the part of the researcher and participant is expected or required to achieve the stated goal of empowerment.

Anderson (1991) acknowledged that intervention by the researcher in the process of research may be seen, by empiricist researchers, as a threat to obtaining valid and reliable data. However, she noted that participants' requests for information, for example, are germane to the research process and are informative regarding how knowledge is produced in social contexts. Further, it was argued by Hall and Stevens (1991) that standards for reliability and validity developed for quantitative research are inappropriate for judging the validity of feminist research, given the relational and contextual nature of women's experiences. They contended that such standards were established to facilitate generalizability, which is based on the assumption of the existence of one reality, and that this assumption is not valid and does not fit the complexity of women's experiences.

Hall and Stevens (1991), in describing rigor in feminist research, argued that the reliability and validity of feminist research should be judged according to criteria whereby the dependability of the research process, the degree of stability of participants' themes over time, and the degree of similarity of responses in a single time period can be affirmed. Further, they stated that the dependability of the research would be strengthened if other researchers were able to construct similar meanings from the raw data, using similar procedures for data analysis and equivalent feminist understandings. They noted that the "more the researcher confirms women's expressive meanings by recurring themes, the greater the accuracy of the data" (p. 24). These meanings can also be validated with the research participants (Campbell & Bunting, 1991; Hall & Stevens, 1991; MacPherson, 1983; Parker & McFarlane, 1991; Thompson, 1991; Webb, 1993) or other groups of women (Hall & Stevens, 1991; MacPherson, 1983), who can, however, provide only an impression of authenticity (Hall & Stevens, 1991).

The search for recurring themes as a measure of accuracy of data is problematic and is indicative of the inconsistency that exists between the epistemology and methodologies that underlie some feminist research. Given an epistemology that holds that no common knowable reality exists and that knowledge is relational and valid only within the context of particular experience, it is contradictory to assume that recurring themes will exist among particular women's experiences. This is because the existence of recurring themes implies that there is a common reality that can be known with regard to the experiences of women. Although the existence of a common reality would be rejected by many feminist theorists, Hall and Stevens (1991) argued that "even though human experiences cannot be generalized, postempiricist researchers assume that some information is transferable from one human context to another" (p. 20). However, it is unclear from their discussion what information is transferable and upon what basis such judgment is made.

Conclusion

Feminist nursing research has made an important contribution to the development of nursing knowledge in that it has provided particular descriptions and explanations of women's experiences that have not been previously available, given the predominant scientific paradigm used in nursing research. Nonetheless, these descriptions and explanations are insufficient, in and of themselves, to direct nursing practice in terms of dealing with the oppression of women. Generalizable descriptive and prescriptive nursing knowledge is required for practice, but problems inherent in the epistemological and methodological underpinnings of feminist research preclude the development of such knowledge. Of primary import, because of all of the implications that flow from it, is the view that there is no reality that exists independent of the mind. Other problems that also must be considered include inconsistencies evident in the epistemological and methodological underpinnings of some feminist research and the blurring of distinctions between research and practice. Unless and until these problems are resolved, nursing practice will remain without the knowledge it requires to deal effectively with women's oppression.

References

Anderson, J. M. (1991). Reflexivity in fieldwork: Toward a feminist epistemology. *Image, 23*, 115-118.

Batey, M. (1991). The research-practice relationship. Response: Research as practice. *Nursing Science Quarterly, 4*(3), 101-103.

Campbell, J. C., & Bunting, S. (1991). Voices and paradigms: Perspectives on critical and feminist theory in nursing. *Advances in Nursing Science, 13*(3), 1-15.

Chinn, P. L. (1981). Women's health. *Advances in Nursing Science, 1*, 1.

Chinn, P. L. (1989). Nursing patterns of knowing and feminist thought. *Nursing and Health Care, 10*(2), 71-75.

Connors, D. D. (1988). A continuum of researcher-participant relationships: An analysis and critique. *Advances in Nursing Science, 10*(4), 32-42.

Doering, L. (1992). Power and knowledge in nursing: A feminist poststructuralist view. *Advances in Nursing Science, 14*(4), 24-33.

Donaldson, S. K., & Crowley, D. M. (1992). The discipline of nursing. In L. H. Nicoll (Ed.), *Perspectives on nursing theory* (2nd ed., pp. 204-215). Philadelphia: J. B. Liiincott. (Original work published 1978)

Duffy, M. (1985). A critique of research: A feminist perspective. *Health Care for Women International, 6,* 341-352.

Dzurec, L. C. (1989). The necessity for and evolution of multiple paradigms for nursing research: A poststructuralist perspective. *Advances in Nursing Science, 11*(4), 69-77.

Hall, J. M., & Stevens, F. E. (1991). Rigor in feminist research. *Advances in Nursing Science, 13*(3), 16-29.

Harding, S. (1987). Introduction: Is there a feminist method? In S. Harding (Ed.), *Feminism and methodology* (pp. 1-14). Bloomington: Indiana University Press.

Kremer, B. (1990). Learning to say no: Keeping feminist research for ourselves. *Women's Studies International Forum, 13,* 463-467.

MacPherson, K. I. (1983). Feminist methods: A new paradigm for nursing research. *Advances in Nursing Science, 5*(1), 17-25.

McBride, A. B. (1984). Nursing and the women's movement. *Image, 16,* 66.

Parker, B., & McFarlane, J. (1991). Feminist theory and nursing: An empowerment model for research. *Advances in Nursing Science, 13*(3), 59-67.

Schultz, R. R., & Meleis, A. I. (1988). Nursing epistemology: Traditions, insights, questions. *Image, 20,* 217-221.

Schumacher, K. L., & Gortner, S. R. (1992). (Mis)conceptions and reconceptions about traditional science. *Advances in Nursing Science, 14*(4), 1-11.

Seibold, C., Richards, L., & Simon, D. (1994). Feminist methodology and qualitative research about midlife. *Journal of Advanced Nursing, 19,* 394-402.

Thompson, J. L. (1991). Exploring gender and culture with Khmer refugee women: Reflections on participatory feminist research. *Advances in Nursing Science, 13*(3), 30-48.

Webb, C. (1984). Feminist methodology in nursing research. *Journal of Advanced Nursing, 9,* 249-256.

Webb, C. (1993). Feminist research: Definitions, methodology, methods, and evaluation. *Journal of Advanced Nursing, 18,* 416-423.

Epilogue: Seeking Truth About Nursing Truth

Having read and considered the preceding chapters, readers in all likelihood will have drawn various conclusions, including the following: (a) Nurses are at least implicitly, operating under a diversity of conceptions of truth in nursing inquiry—some conceptions being contrary to others; (b) nurses have begun to reject traditional conceptions of truth that focus on objective truth and to adopt those that focus on subjective truth and the meaningful; and (c) there is a growing urgency to sort out what is true about nursing truth—at minimum, to determine the kinds, measures, and expressions of truth that are appropriate in nursing inquiry. All of these developments warrant our attention and study; the future of the nursing discipline depends on it. It would seem that action taken on the third development—the growing need to seek what is true about nursing truth—would provide us with the knowledge we require to deal with the other two. It would help us determine whether we should be promoting them and, if not, the course we should take instead.

If we were able to come to some agreement about which kinds, measures, and expressions of truth are appropriate in nursing inquiry, then we would have the beginning of a conception of nursing truth—a conception that, when fully developed, would hold the potential to unite nurse researchers, theorists, scholars, practitioners, and educators in their efforts to improve nursing practice. Without an adequate conception of nursing truth, our efforts at nursing knowledge development are bound to continue to "be all over the place," with the end result being the likely demise of the nursing discipline.

What, then, would the pursuit of truth about nursing truth entail? For one thing, it would require that we make up our minds about such basic matters as the nature of reality, the nature of human cognitive powers of knowing, and the nature of truth and knowledge. Either reality is knowable or it is not. Either humans can attain objective knowledge or they cannot. Either knowledge is a matter of truth or it is not. Common sense would say that we cannot have it both ways. Yet it would seem that some nurse theorists must think otherwise when they claim that reality is unknowable, that attainment of objective knowledge is impossible, or that falsity and error are irrelevant matters in the attainment of knowledge. Surely, in their everyday lives, they do not find themselves operating under such beliefs.

It is hard to see how anyone could survive for very long functioning in terms of the belief that humans cannot come to know reality as it exists independent of the mind and cannot attain objective knowledge of it. Operating thus in everyday matters, would we not soon meet our end (e.g., in motor vehicular traffic)? Would others not soon meet with disaster at our hands in nursing practice? Why, then, do these nurse theorists hold so tenaciously to the beliefs that they do, when functioning in terms of them would have the most dire effects?

Could it be that they do not see the contradiction involved? Could it be that they see the contradiction but are not bothered by it because, in their minds, contradiction is not a problem? Could it be that they see the contradiction, are bothered by it, and are searching for ways to deal with the problem? Are recent publications, such as those by Packard and Polifroni (1992) and by Wolfer (1993), reflective of the recognition, by some nurse scholars, of this very need? Or could it be simply a matter of preoccupation with making room for subjective aspects of truth in nursing inquiry and practice? Are the new ways of inquiry that are being developed in qualitative research indicative of efforts to supplement or infuse the purely objective with "heart"—somehow to make room for the feeling, the meaningful, the creative, and the subjective (all of which common sense would say are essential in nursing practice)?

Regardless of what motive force is operative, it is clear from the essays in this volume (as well as from other nursing literature) that a diversity of conceptions of the nature of reality, of humans, and of truth and knowledge prevail in the nurse's world. To help us make up our minds about these basic matters, we would suggest that nurse scholars collectively determine through disciplined discussion (a) what is being presupposed—held to be true—about these matters in existing conceptions of nursing (and of nursing truth) and (b) the implications of those presuppositions for nursing thought and action, in light of common sense. By so doing, we would increase the likelihood of obtaining agreement on matters foundational and integral to seeking what is true about nursing truth—to developing an adequate conception of nursing truth. It would be expected that at bare minimum, the kinds, measures, and expressions of truth appropriate in nursing inquiry would be identified in that conception.

In addition, if we are to succeed in developing an adequate conception of nursing truth, we must be prepared to ask critical, generative questions, such as those included among the "Guiding Questions" in this volume, about existing conceptions of nursing (and of nursing truth). For example, suppose that in a particular conception, it is claimed that (a) what is true for you may not be true for me and that (b) nursing practice ought to be based on nursing's body of knowledge. Then an answer sought to the following question would be generative of vital developments: "If truth is a subjective matter, leaving no place for error or falsity, then would nursing acts, based on nursing's body of knowledge, always be error free?" Or suppose, in another conceptualization, it is claimed that (a) truth is immutable and that (b) nursing truths ought to reflect changes in nursing practice. Then questions such as the following might be asked: "If truth is immutable, then how can nursing truths reflect changes in nursing practice?"

All too often, when a conception of truth seems to be wanting, we do not do anything about it. Sometimes it is simply because we think we probably have not understood it. If this is the case, then we ought to put forth sincere effort to come to understand it. That done, if we still find it wanting, then we are called upon to enter into collegial discussion of it. As we all know, making that happen is easier said than done. Nonetheless, we must try.

It is not only interesting but significant to note that despite the popular claim that truth is unattainable, most people, including nurses, continue to seek truth about truth. At the conference at which the essays in this volume were presented, it was clearly evident that a good number of the nurse participants were skeptical about the matter of examining the veridical and deceptive aspects of conceptions of truth regnant in nursing thought. What is remarkable is that these nurses nonetheless had made the effort to attend the conference, knowing it would focus on that very topic.

Perhaps, despite our skeptical claims, we continue to search for an adequate definition of truth and of nursing truth because we realize, at some level, that our sanity depends on it (not to mention the possibility of our being able to work cooperatively for the betterment of humankind). If that is so, we have much to gain from continuing to seek truth about nursing truth and much to lose from not doing so.

References

Packard, S. A., & Polifroni, E. C. (1992). The nature of scientific truth. *Nursing Science Quarterly, 5*(4), 158-163.

Wolfer, J. (1993). Aspects of "reality" and ways of knowing in nursing: In search of an integrating paradigm. *Image, 25*(2), 141-146.

Index

About the Editors

June F. Kikuchi, RN, PhD, holds the positions of Professor and Director of the Institute for Philosophical Nursing Research (IPNR) at the University of Alberta, Faculty of Nursing, Edmonton, Alberta. She received a BScN from the University of Toronto and an MN and a PhD in nursing from the University of Pittsburgh. Postdoctorally, she studied philosophy at the University of Toronto. She is the Co-Founder of the IPNR. She has published papers on philosophic nursing inquiry, nursing knowledge development, and the quality of life of children of disabled parents. She has presented papers nationally and internationally on those topics as well as on the development of nursing research in health care agencies. She is the coeditor of the IPNR conference publications *Philosophic Inquiry in Nursing* and *Developing a Philosophy of Nursing.*

Donna M. Romyn, RN, MN, is a Lecturer at the University of Alberta, Faculty of Nursing, Edmonton, Alberta. She holds a BScN and an MN from the University of Alberta and is completing her PhD studies in nursing at that university. Her dissertation entails a philosophical analysis of feminist and critical pedagogies in nursing education. Of late, she has been involved in nursing education program development and evaluation. Her presentations and publications have focused on Roy's and Orem's conceptualizations of nursing, nursing education, nursing management of pain, data sharing, and secondary data analysis.

Helen Simmons, PhD, is an Associate Professor and the Associate Director and Co-Founder of the Institute for Philosophical Nursing Research (IPNR) at the University of Alberta, Faculty of Nursing, Edmonton, Alberta. She received a BA in psychology and philosophy and an MA in clinical psychology from the University of British Columbia and a PhD in educational psychology from the University of Oregon. She has pursued postdoctoral studies in philosophy at the Aspen Institute for Humanistic Studies. Her publications and presentations have focused on health, public health, philosophic nursing inquiry, and nursing knowledge development. She is the coeditor of the IPNR conference publications *Philosophic Inquiry in Nursing* and *Developing a Philosophy of Nursing.* She was awarded an honorary life membership in the Alberta Association of Registered Nurses for her contributions to the nursing profession.

About the Contributors

Anne H. Bishop, RN, EdD, is a Professor at Lynchburg College, Department of Nursing, Lynchburg, Virginia. She received a BSN, an MSN, and an EdD from the University of Virginia and an MEd from Lynchburg College. She is well known for her work with philosopher John R. Scudder Jr., with whom she has coauthored several books and articles in the areas of nursing practice, caring, ethics, and phenomenology. Their recently published book, *The Practical, Moral and Personal Sense of Nursing: A Phenomenological Philosophy of Practice,* is being read and cited internationally.

Robyn J. Holden, RPN, PhD, holds the position of Associate Professor in the Medical Research Unit at the University of Wollongong, New South Wales, Australia. She is a recipient of a BA degree with three majors in sociology, philosophy, and psychology from La Trobe University, an honors degree in psychology from the University of Wollongong, and an MA and a PhD in philosophical studies from Deakin University. She also holds a diploma in applied science (advanced psychiatric nursing) from the Phillip Institute of Technology. She serves on the editorial board of *Holistic Nursing Practice* and the *Australian and New Zealand Journal of Mental Health Nursing* and is a member of the review panel of *Contemporary Nurse.* Her research and publi-

cations in the areas of neuropsychiatric and neurodegenerative disor-
ders and nursing theory are gaining international recognition.

Joy L. Johnson, RN, PhD, is an Assistant Professor at the University
of British Columbia, School of Nursing, Vancouver, British Columbia.
She holds a diploma in critical care nursing and a BScN from the
University of British Columbia and an MN and a PhD in nursing from
the University of Alberta. She has been awarded numerous academic
scholarships—most recently, a postdoctoral fellowship to conduct
research in the area of health promotion. She is the author, coauthor,
and coeditor of major publications in the areas of nursing as art and
science, qualitative research, and health promotion.

Shirley Cloutier Laffrey, RN, PhD, is an Associate Professor at the
University of Texas at Austin, School of Nursing. She earned a diploma
in nursing at St. Joseph Hospital School of Nursing and in public
health at McGill University, a BSN and a PhD in nursing at Wayne
State University, and an MPH at the University of Michigan. Her
long-standing interest in community health nursing and health promotion is evident in and pervades all aspects of her work. More
recently, her research publications have focused on the health of the
elderly and outcomes of community health nursing with the elderly.

Joy Hinson Penticuff, RN, PhD, FAAN, holds the positions of Associate Professor and of Assistant Dean (Academic Programs) at the
University of Texas at Austin, School of Nursing. She received a BSN
from the Medical College of Georgia and an MSN and a PhD in
clinical psychology from Case Western Reserve University. She has
served as a Postdoctoral Fellow in the Centre for Ethics, Baylor
College of Medicine. She is the recipient of several academic and
professional awards. On many occasions she has served as a consult-
ant, presented papers, and published in her research areas of interest
of ethics and neonatal/perinatal nursing practice.

Lynn Rew, RN, EdD, FAAN, is an Associate Professor at the University
of Texas at Austin, School of Nursing. She earned a BSN from the
University of Hawaii and an MSN and an EdD at Northern Illinois

University. She is a Founding Member of the American Holistic Nurses' Association, has held various professional executive positions, and has received many scholarly awards. Her research areas of interest and expertise, in which she has published numerous papers, include nursing/nurses' intuition, psychiatric/mental health nursing, and child/adolescent sexual abuse. She is currently a Postdoctoral Fellow in the Adolescent Health Program, School of Medicine, University of Minnesota.

Margarete J. Sandelowski, RN, PhD, FAAN, is a Professor at the University of North Carolina at Chapel Hill, School of Nursing. She holds a diploma in nursing from Beth Israel Hospital School of Nursing, a BSN from the University of Pennsylvania, an MS in maternal-child nursing from Boston University, an EdM from Columbia University Teachers College, and a PhD in American Studies from Case Western Reserve University. She has published extensively in nursing and social science journals and anthologies on the subjects of reproductive technology, technology in nursing, infertility, and qualitative methods. She is the author of several books, including *With Child in Mind: Studies of the Personal Encounter With Infertility,* which was awarded the 1994 Eileen Basker Memorial Prize. She is currently working on a social history of technology in nursing.

Rozella M. Schlotfeldt, RN, PhD, FAAN, holds the position of Professor Emeritus and Dean Emeritus at Case Western Reserve University, School of Nursing, Cleveland, Ohio. She received a BS in nursing from the University of Iowa and an MS in nursing education/administration and a PhD in education curriculum development from the University of Chicago. She holds several honorary doctoral degrees as well as many other significant awards. She is recognized and respected nationally and internationally for her substantial contributions to the development of the nursing profession, particularly in the areas of nursing education and nursing knowledge development, in which she has presented papers and published widely. She has served in numerous locales as a visiting professor and has held a wide variety of prominent offices within nursing organizations.

Jean Watson, RN, PhD, FAAN, is a Distinguished Professor of Nursing and the Founder and Director of the Center for Human Caring at the University of Colorado, Health Sciences Center, Denver, Colorado. She earned a diploma in nursing at the Lewis-Gale School of Nursing and a BS in nursing, an MS in psychiatric-mental health nursing, and a PhD in educational psychology and counseling at the University of Colorado. Her published works on the philosophy and theory of human caring and the art and science of nursing are used throughout the world. She is the recipient of various prestigious awards and honors, including two honorary doctoral degrees. More recently, she has held a Kellogg Fellowship in Australia and a Fulbright Research Award in Sweden. She has served as Distinguished Lecturer and Endowed Lecturer at universities in the United States and abroad.